Removing Processed Food From Your Life

Trudi Hemstrong

Section I:

Ultra-Processed & Processed Foods, Sugar & Health

Introduction

Welcome! *Removing Processed Food From Your Life* is a concise but complete resource for people who would like to limit or eliminate the most harmful foods and drinks from their diet, which are ultra-processed foods and sugar.

Section I. of *Removing Processed Food From Your Life* gives you an in-depth review of the ways in which processed foods, especially ultra-processed foods and drinks as well as sugar, affect every part of the human body, including the brain, heart, and liver. We'll discuss why processed and especially ultra-processed foods and sugar are **highly addictive** in the ways they affect the human brain.

We will also address how processed foods/drinks and sugar drive insulin resistance, which now affects 88% of American adults, most without knowing it. Insulin resistance causes prediabetes and Type 2 diabetes, drives weight gain & obesity, hypertension, and cholesterol problems such as high triglycerides. It's what's been *done* to our food—i.e. making it highly refined and processed—that's driving these serious problems with our hormone insulin as a population and driving addiction to these foods.

We don't necessarily think of food affecting our hormones so directly and profoundly, but in fact what we eat and drink is the single most important factor influencing insulin, which is the chief hormone in the human body.

Insulin regulates blood sugar and fat storage among so many other jobs in the human body. The "calories" in ultra- and processed foods are not the primary issue. The most important issue is *how* all the highly refined ingredients in ultra- and processed foods/drinks and sugar directly affect our hormones, biochemistry, cardiovascular system, and especially our brain chemistry.

We'll discuss why refining and processing foods *fundamentally alters* how the entire human body responds to them. Adding sugar, fats, chemicals, salt, flavorings and other substances makes these foods exceptionally attractive to humans for reasons that are evolutionary in origin, not individual or personal.

We'll discuss these reasons so you can better understand why cravings for these foods are so powerful and why they're now the majority of the American diet.

We'll begin by using the *NOVA* classification system to discuss the differences between **unprocessed**, **processed**, and **ultra-processed foods/drinks** so you can focus on making the best choices about what to consume and what to avoid. The key to removing processed and especially ultra-processed foods and drinks from your life, including sugar, and eliminating the cravings for these foods is preparing your own meals and snacks.

The fast food and processed food industries spend *a lot of money* making us believe it's too time-consuming and complicated to prepare and cook our own meals; *this is not true!*

Section II of *Removing Processed Food From Your Life* is a practical manual and detailed guide to shopping for, prepping, and cooking a full week's worth of fantastic, delicious, healthy meals. You will learn how to prepare and cook *7 days of breakfasts, lunches, and dinners, by spending only 2 hours total in the kitchen each week*.

The comprehensive shopping list provided in *Removing Processed Food From Your Life* means you shop once a week, saving both time and money. This list also helps you avoid impulse purchases and processed foods when you shop.

When we remove ultra- and processed foods/drinks as well as sugar from our lives and shop for the meals and healthy snacks we're going to prepare each week, we also save a lot of money.

The reason we save money is because although processed and ultra-processed foods/drinks, including fast food and prepared meals, *appear* to cost less than healthy, whole foods, they are actually far more expensive in several ways, both directly and in the long term.

Thus, the key to successfully removing ultra- and processed foods/drinks and sugar from your life, saving money, and saving time, is preparing your own meals and snacks so that you always have plenty of healthy and natural foods available at home and to take with you.

Section II of this book, "Shopping, Organizing, and Preparing Food" gives you a detailed list of staple foods that are the foundation of a healthy, unprocessed diet that will leave you satisfied and significantly reduce the cravings for ultra-processed foods and sugar.

Section II guides you, step-by-step, through preparing and cooking a week's worth of meals in 2 hours because preparing your own meals and snacks makes it *much* easier to make healthy food choices on a daily basis.

Healthy, convenient meals are what allow us to remove ultra-processed foods/drinks and sugar from our lives and improve our health significantly. This is why the ultra- and processed food and sugar industries want you to believe the *myth* that we're far too busy to prepare our own meals.

If you can set aside 2 hours a week, either at one time or for 1 hour twice a week, you *can* have 7 days of breakfasts ready to just reheat in the microwave while you're getting ready for your day, lunches packed and ready to take with you, and dinners waiting for you when you get home after a busy day.

For example, breakfast becomes a matter of quickly reheating a delicious, filling omelet, or a wonderful bowl of slow-cooked whole oatmeal in the microwave, yogurt with berries, nuts and seeds—everything already made. Lunches are a feast already prepared in individual containers that you just grab from the fridge and take with you on your way out the door.

When you come home tired from work, dinner is only a matter of getting a plate and choosing from a wide range of meat and fish, vegetables, grains, and other delicious choices that are already prepared and waiting for you. Thus, dinner every night *is much faster* than ordering takeout, getting fast food, or stopping at the store for a pre-prepared meal.

Best of all, throughout the week there's no food prep, no cooking, no cleaning up cooking dishes, etc. Two hours per week gives you 21 meals—and you'll save money too. We'll discuss how to do all of this in Section II of this book. *It is* a lot easier than you think!

We will discuss the following health issues in detail in Section I of *Removing Processed Food From Your Life* as part of helping you understand why processed foods and drinks affect us, particularly our brains, very differently than other foods, but there's a few things to keep in mind about these foods.

The ingredients in ultra-and processed foods/drinks are simple, usually refined grains, starches, sugars, and "vegetable" oils. They add flavorings, and fabricate them into different shapes and foods, so it seems like there's endless variety of these foods. There isn't.

It's all the same incredibly cheap ingredients, so the profit margins are extremely high. This is why companies spend billions of dollars in advertising, *not on the ingredients in these foods*, ingredients that disproportionately harm human health for reasons we'll discuss.

These foods are *intentionally* designed and manufactured to be addictive; these foods are highly addictive for reasons that lie in our evolutionary history as humans, including how these foods affect the reward centers of the human brain.

We'll also discuss why the *refined ingredients* in these foods, *not the calories*, are what adversely affect our hormones and drive problems with weight, blood sugar, blood pressure, and other chronic health problems.

What are the costs of processed and ultra-processed foods and drinks? The costs are significant, both in terms of money and our health. Ultra-processed foods and drinks, *which now comprise the majority of the American diet*, have little to no nutritional value.

This means we're spending a lot of money on foods and drinks, including most prepared meals, that give us calories and raise blood sugar so we think, temporarily, that we're satisfied; however, given what's in them, these substances don't nourish us or provide our bodies with the healthy macro- and micronutrients we must have. They're not just expensive, "empty" calories, they're costly toxic and addictive calories.

Processed and ultra-processed foods make us feel, briefly, that we're full by spiking our blood sugar significantly. However, when our blood sugar drops again just as dramatically, we become *even hungrier* and crave the ultra-and processed foods and drinks that will spike blood sugar again. This cycle gets worse over time, which leads to insulin resistance.

This is a key reason cravings for processed foods and sugar worsen and can be difficult to control—i.e. it's because of the ways in which these substances cause extreme spikes and drops in blood sugar.

Very often we don't realize this is happening at all, but the cravings are a prominent sign this is what's going on. Processed and ultra-processed foods are *designed* to do this to our blood sugar so we'll keep eating them while never feeling satisfying as blood sugar and insulin levels get worse in response.

We'll discuss why *un*processed foods actually *decrease* hunger and appetite, reduce cravings substantially, and work properly with our blood sugar, hormones, genes, biochemistry, and neurochemistry.

We'll talk about why ultra-processed foods and drinks are designed and formulated to *manipulate* our biochemistry, hormones, and neurochemistry.

They cause serious metabolic diseases and conditions such as Type 2 diabetes, weight gain, hypertension, nonalcoholic fatty liver disease (NAFLD), cardiovascular disease, and dementia among many other chronic health problems.

This means ultra-processed foods and drinks are extremely expensive in terms of their costs to our health. This includes all the medications a majority of American adults must now use to "treat" the chronic conditions and diseases *these foods cause over time.*

This means we're paying for these ultra-processed foods/drinks with our health, expensive medications, lost productivity, and lower quality of life. The vast majority of our chronic health problems as a society are due to diet-driven diseases and conditions rooted in processed and ultra-processed foods and drinks. These now represent *75% of all healthcare costs.* These include Type 2 diabetes, high blood pressure, NAFLD, weight problems, and cholesterol problems.

These "foods" also drive cardiovascular disease and dementia because of the ways in which these foods affect blood sugar and the hormone insulin, which we'll address.

Ultra-processed (and many processed) foods and drinks are highly addictive to humans, especially sugar. These foods are addictive because they're formulated to be addictive; the addictive nature of these foods and drinks is *intentional.*

Not everyone becomes addicted to them, but given that these "foods" now comprise the majority of our diet in the U.S., and increasingly across the globe, addiction is very widespread, and it's getting worse. It's not that we lack willpower as a species; we're being exposed to these foods and drinks *everywhere* as a population and in all age groups.

These addictive "foods" are *normalized* in the culture in ways that other addictive substances such as cigarettes, alcohol, and a wide range of addictive drugs are not normalized or available in our everyday lives in all environments.

Ultra-processed and many processed foods are addictive in the ways that tobacco products and many drugs are addictive because ultra-processed foods and drinks *affect the same regions of the brain* as these other toxic, addictive substances do—*but they do so even more quickly* than many of these drugs and substances.

The manufacturers know this science; they know exactly what they're doing, and it's legal. Thus a very costly aspect of ultra-processed foods and drinks, especially sugar, is addiction or potential addiction, addiction that is *normalized and promoted* in so many environments.

We must be clear that these substances are *inherently* addictive, because they're *made* to be addictive just as cigarettes and a wide range of drugs are. The issue is not failure of willpower or personal weakness; these are the ways in which this massive social and cultural problem with our food supply is made to *seem* like a matter of individual, personal failure.

Processed and especially ultra-processed foods and drinks put anyone who consumes them at risk of addiction for reasons that have to do with how the human brain works, how our ancient hormonal system works, and because of the way we evolved over millions of years as a species.

These foods and drinks are *created* to target our evolutionary vulnerabilities for sweet and refined foods, manipulate our brain chemistry, and foster intense cravings via rollercoaster blood sugar—because its profitable to do so, *very* profitable.

Thus, processed foods—especially ultra-processed foods and drinks—affect the human brain, our blood sugar, and our hormones in profound ways—biochemical effects we *do not control* through willpower, or personal choice, or reducing calories, etc.—i.e. all the excuses we're given about why these foods aren't the problem when they *are the problem*.

All ultra-processed foods and sugar are toxic; they are not food. Limiting or eliminating incredibly harmful ultra-processed foods and drinks, especially those that contain sugar, takes time. It's a process that necessitates replacing these substances with whole and natural foods and drinks.

Therefore, ensuring these ultra-processed foods and drinks *are not available in your home*, is crucial. Think of these "foods" as substances to which one is exposed. We reduce or eliminate exposure to toxic substances in our homes, including dangerous chemicals.

We need to do this with our food supply as a society, but given that these substances are legal, we can begin by getting these toxins out of our homes and meals. Section II of this book will guide you in making this process much easier.

Given that ultra-processed foods and drinks, especially sugar, affect our brain chemistry very differently than unprocessed foods, often we consume ultra-processed foods and drinks in response to stressors such as sadness, boredom, fear, anxiety— as well as to celebrate occasions.

Thus, given the strong links between ultra-processed foods, drinks, and sugar and our complex emotional lives, it's crucial to ensure that these foods are not accessible in your home—and that you have many healthy alternatives from which to choose.

The ultra-processed food/drink and sugar industries also want you to believe that the profound damage their toxic substances cause (remember, they're not food) to every aspect of human health isn't related to their products.

They want you to believe our widespread chronic, diet-driven health problems, conditions, and diseases are caused by people eating too many "calories" and "burning" too few. This is total bull, to put it bluntly.

The science is very clear, but these companies spend enormous amounts of money making false equivalences such "all calories are equal", we need to "burn" more "energy" than we consume, etc., when the human body *does not* work this way. The human body has no receptors for "calories." When we put something in our mouths, our bodies do very complex things with these foods and drinks, which we'll discuss.

However, adding up and subtracting calories *is not* what human cells, genes, or hormones do! We can add and subtract, but our bodies can't—and it's very important to remember this when you hear nonsense that "all calories are equal." The processed food and beverage giants *want* you to focus on the wrong thing, calories, so you will internalize and blame yourself for the toxic effects of *their* substances.

Weight gain is primarily a hormonal imbalance issue. The foods/drinks we consume largely determine how our hormones behave. However, it's the carbohydrate, protein, and fat in these foods—*and the degree of their refinement—not their "calories—"* that affect our hormonal system and cause hormonal imbalances, especially insulin resistance, which causes weight gain. We'll go into how this works in detail.

Exercise is important for many reasons, but it has very little to do with managing weight. Calories are not the issue when it comes to our health and weight for reasons we'll discuss.

It's *the way* ultra-processed foods/drinks and sugar affect our hormones that is the single biggest driver of the chronic metabolic health problems facing us today, including obesity, prediabetes and Type 2 diabetes, hypertension, and cholesterol problems—specifically high triglycerides.

Therefore, significantly limiting or eliminating consumption of ultra-processed foods and drinks is the *single most important thing you can do for every aspect of your health*. Nothing else comes close in terms of improving your health, now and for the future.

Again, exercise is absolutely wonderful for us; physical movement relieves stress, releases chemicals in our bodies and brains that improve mood, strengthens our muscles, including our hearts, improves brain functioning, and affects gene expression among many other powerful benefits.

Exercise for all these wonderful benefits, but don't focus on "burning" calories. Exercise helps us lose weight *because it helps insulin work far better in our bodies*. when insulin is working properly in our bodies, two things happen: 1.) we store less fat and 2.) our cells release more fatty acids (i.e. lose weight).

This entire process is hormonal and has nothing to do with calories. Given that ultra- and processed foods and drinks, especially sugar, are what drive problems with insulin in the first place, removing these foods and drinks from your life to the degree you can is the *direct route* to controlling weight.

Getting enough daily exercise, such as 30-minute walk each day, is also a very powerful way to reduce cravings for ultra-processed foods / drinks—because of the ways in which exercise positively affects our neurochemistry.

You don't have to exercise in ways that aren't feasible or too demanding for your body; remember, this is not about "burning calories."

Exercise is about improving your health, including your brain health and the health of your hormonal system.
The hormones leptin (appetite/satiety) and insulin (fat storage / growth factor / blood sugar regulation) work properly in response to a diet of primarily unprocessed and minimally processed foods.

When these two powerful hormones are working properly they *stabilize* appetite and cravings for processed foods and sugar go down significantly. It's the refined and processed nature of ultra-processed foods in particular that causes such havoc with our hormones.

To summarize, ultra-processed foods/drinks and sugar are *not food*. They are toxic substances. They have little to no nutritional value, and the nutritional requirement for sugar in the human diet is zero. Ultra-processed foods and drinks are highly addictive because they're *designed* to be addictive, and they are ubiquitous in our food environments, and we're *encouraged* in myriad ways to make them central to our lives.

These substances affect our metabolic health in profound ways, including our blood sugar and the powerful hormone insulin, which is our fat storage hormone.

The manufacturers of these substances do everything they can to get us to believe we're dependent on these foods because it's too time-consuming and difficult to prepare our own meals, when that is just not true. Two hours per week in the kitchen ensures you have an entire week of amazing meals.

The makers of ultra-processed foods and drinks want us to believe that the epidemic of chronic health problems, including weight problems, Type 2 diabetes, and hypertension, isn't due to their toxic, addictive substances affecting our cardiovascular system and brains and hormones, especially insulin.

They want us to believe the entrenched myth that all the chronic metabolic health problems that now affect the majority of Americans are due to consuming too many calories and burning too few—i.e. to our "choices." The problem is, this explanation defies both science and logic.

The powerful hormone insulin is especially important in relation to ultra-processed foods and drinks because these substances cause **insulin resistance** over time. Insulin resistance causes prediabetes and Type 2 diabetes, weight problems, most cases of hypertension, cholesterol problems, Metabolic Syndrome, and dementia. Nonalcoholic fatty liver disease (NAFLD) and cardiovascular disease are tied to insulin resistance as well.

Essentially the vast majority of our health problems as a population are due to one thing: ultra-processed foods/drinks and sugar. These substances are behind 75% of all healthcare costs in the U.S. and increasingly around the globe.

Let's get started by examining the differences between whole/natural foods, processed foods/drinks, and ultra-processed foods and drinks. *It's important to note that what we drink is as important as what we eat.* In some cases that we'll discuss, what we drink has even more harmful consequences for our health and for driving cravings.

Understanding Ultra-Processed Foods/Drinks and Sugar; What Are They?

First, let's discuss the important differences between **whole and natural foods, processed foods, and ultra-processed foods/drinks.**

It's helpful to use the *NOVA* food classification system to understand the differences between natural, processed, and ultra-processed foods/drinks. You can find a good summary of this classification system in *World Nutrition*.[1] A shorter summary is available in *Public Health Nutrition*, a journal published by Cambridge University Press.

The main concept to understand when it comes to what we eat and drink is that "the most salient division of foods and drinks is in terms of their type, degree and purpose of processing."[2] I strongly encourage you to follow the hyperlinks above and read more about this classification system of food processing.

Here is a summary of the *NOVA* classification of foods. (Please note I've omitted one category in order to focus on these 3 principle categories):

Unprocessed or Minimally Processed Foods are the edible parts of plants, animals, and fungi after separation from nature.

---

[1] *World Nutrition*, Vol 7, No. 1-3: January-March, 2016: http://archive.wphna.org/wp-content/uploads/2016/01/WN-2016-7-1-3-28-38-Monteiro-Cannon-Levy-et-al-NOVA.pdf

[2] *Public Health Nutrition*, Volume 12, Issue 5 , May 2009, pp. 729 – 731. DOI: https://doi.org/10.1017/S1368980009005291

These are minimally processed foods that remove inedible or unwanted parts (stems, seeds, leaves, organs/bones, dirt, etc.); the processing in this category is to extend the life of these unprocessed foods.

Examples include meat, poultry, eggs, milk, mushrooms, whole vegetables and fruits, legumes and beans, grains such as brown rice and quinoa, etc. *None of these processes adds substances such as sugar, oils, fats, salt, flavorings, etc.*

Processed Foods: These are simple products made by adding sugar, oil, salt, and most of these foods have very few ingredients. These include canned vegetables, fruits, and legumes, salted or sugared nuts and seeds, smoked/cured meats, canned fish and meats, cheeses, unpackaged and freshly made breads.

Ultra-processed Foods and Drinks, the ultra processed category, is the one that predicts morbidity and mortality, and is 56% of the food and 62% of the sugar consumed in the United States. These are **industrially created and produced** and often contain multiple ingredients including sugar, oils, fats, salt, stabilizers, preservatives, etc.

These "foods" now constitute **nearly 60% of the American diet**, which is an astronomical increase in just a few decades. Many of the ingredients are substances that you won't find in normal culinary preparation—i.e. stuff you don't use at home when you cook.

Substances found only in ultra-processed products include things such as casein, lactose, whey, gluten, hydrogenated oils, hydrolyzed proteins, soy protein isolate, maltodextrin, high fructose corn syrup, dyes, stabilizers, flavor enhancers, and processing aids such as anti-bulking, de-foaming, anti-caking, and glazing agents, emulsifiers, and humectants.

Ultra-processed foods and drinks also use many non-sugar sweeteners; these also spike blood sugar and insulin levels, drive fatty liver disease, cause weight gain, and increase inflammation in the body and brain, which profoundly affects our hearts. The fact that these non-sugar sweeteners may not have "calories" is *entirely* beside the point; the substantial damage these substances to our bodies do has nothing to do with "calories."

These products **are created and fabricated using processes that have no equivalent in home preparation such as extrusion, moulding, etc.** A key characteristic of ultra-processed foods and drinks is that they have an incredible amount of sugar. Many also use "alternative" sweeteners such as honey and agave as well as artificial sweeteners, which harm our health, raise insulin levels, and promote weight gain.

These ultra-processed "foods" and drinks are very often uniform. If you buy the product in one supermarket it will be exactly the same in another supermarket, convenience store, big box store, etc. Ultra-processed foods and drinks are all about uniformity, shelf stability, transportation needs, and most especially, profits—including juices and drinks that claim to be healthy.

Keep in mind that manufacturers use terms such as "all natural," "plant-based," and "healthy" to sell us ultra-processed foods and drinks that destroy our health and foster addiction and cravings.

They use colors, type fonts, labeling, advertising strategies, shelving positions, celebrity endorsements, product placements and many other techniques to get us to believe these ultra-processed substances are not toxic, that they're "convenient," and that they will fulfill emotional or other needs.

Increasingly processed food companies are using green washing to portray their ultra-processed substances as better for the planet. All the science tells us this is not the case.

Ultra-processed foods and drinks are made with the very cheapest ingredients possible; the manufacturers spend billions in advertising, *not on what goes into these "foods" and drinks.* They're comprised of very few things: **highly refined grains, starches, and sugars, including fructose, along with chemicals and "vegetable" oils such as soybean and canola oils.**

These few "ingredients" in ultra-processed foods and drinks are incredibly cheap, and they can be processed and fabricated into endless shapes and textures and colors to make them *appear* to be different "foods" and drinks. It's all same toxic ingredients.

It's also important to keep in mind that sugar is added to 74% of packaged foods in supermarkets[3]—even if the list of Ingredients doesn't list "sugar" or lists it farther down on the list—it's there under all kinds of other names. Often we don't know we're consuming high levels of sugar in so many forms because manufacturers use *hide sugar behind* **more than 260+ names.** [4]

Many seemingly "healthy" foods such as breakfast bars, cereals and other products that are touted as "whole grain" contain huge amounts of sugar in many forms. These "whole grain" products are almost all ultra-processed and refined, no matter what the packaging says.

Hiding sugar like this is legal, and manufacturers use more than 260 complicated terms to deliberately hide sugar and sweeteners in the Nutrition Fact labels.

---

[3] *Hidden In Plain Sight.* In *Sugarscience*: *The Unsweetened* Truth. University of California San Franscisco: **https://sugarscience.ucsf.edu/hidden-in-plain-sight/**

[4] Hypoglycemia Support Foundation. "US Sugar Consumption, 1822-2005." **https://hypoglycemia.org/added-sugar-repository/**

But all these sources of sugar and sweeteners cause serious harm to the body. For example, we don't necessarily identify these things as sugar that harm our health, but they are: dextrin; dextrose; glucose solids; maltodextrin, maltol; mannose; panocha, etc.

Manufacturers reverse engineer ultra-processed "foods" and drinks—i.e. they start with what how they want the Nutrition Fact labels and Ingredient lists to appear to consumers, so people will think these "foods" and drinks are not as toxic as they are.

Then they fabricate the "food" or drink itself—hiding the sugar and sweeteners under terms they know people aren't going to look up.
We don't bring a biochemistry textbook to the store in order to understand what's in a box of crackers, or an "energy" drink, a jarred tomato sauces, or a supposedly healthy "whole grain" product, etc.

All these 260+ sweeteners, whether they're included in the grams of "added sugar" or not, profoundly affect blood sugar, insulin secretion, weight, blood pressure, cardiovascular, and brain health.

In addition to obvious ultra-processed foods and drinks such as candies, cakes, pies, ice cream, sodas, pastries and desserts of any sort, ultra-processed foods and drinks include pre-packaged salty/savory foods such as chips, pretzels, and crackers.

Although these savory or salty foods don't seem sweet, they have a lot of added sweeteners in them too—often hidden under various names.

Like sweet ultra-processed foods, salty or savory snacks and foods also metabolize very quickly into sugar in the human body because they're made with the cheapest refined grains and starches and sugars and toxic oils, so they spike blood sugar and insulin response; even if they don't seem to have a lot of "added" sugar, to the human body, *they are sugar.*

All this extra sugar (glucose) these ultra-processed foods and drinks become in the human body, whether these products taste sweet or salty, has to go somewhere if we're not using all this glucose for constant physical movement all day.

All this excess glucose beyond our actual energy needs ends up getting stored as fat on our bodies and *in our organs* such as the liver and pancreas gland.

Finally, ultra-processed foods and drinks also include **all** mass-produced breads and buns, margarines and spreads, **all** breakfast cereals, energy bars and drinks, salad dressings and marinades, all processed drinks, milk drinks, fruit yogurts, instant sauces, all soda and nearly all juices, etc.

Ultra-processed foods/drinks also includes infant formulas and other baby products, fortified or powdered meal substitutes, ready-to-eat product such as pies, pasta dishes, pizza, chicken, fish and meat "nuggets" and "sticks," burgers, hot dogs, and other reconstituted meat products as well as "instant" soups and noodles, etc.

In other words, when you're buying something in a package, bag, or in a jar with a barcode, *it's very likely that it's ultra-processed.* When you buy meat, seafood, etc. that's minimally processed, they package it and put a barcode on it at the meat or seafood counter, but it's not an ultra-processed food with all the added sugar, salt, oils, etc.

If you buy meat/seafood that has added flavors and marinades, then you're getting the salt, sugar, oils, and other harmful ingredients.

The above categories, **natural/unprocessed foods, processed foods, and ultra-processed foods/drinks**, are the categories to use when making choices about what to eat and drink. The more we eat and drink foods and beverages from the **natural /unprocessed foods category**, the better.

These are primarily foods that don't come in a package or jar such as whole vegetables, fruits, genuinely whole grains such as quinoa, and nuts and seeds without flavors, sugar, salt, etc.

It's eating and drinking **items in category # 3, ultra-processed foods and drinks**, which **include most restaurant meals and prepared foods,** that causes the vast majority of diet-driven health problems, food addictions and cravings.

It's these "foods" that increase appetite as well as evade and manipulate our appetite and satiety hormone **leptin** so we genuinely don't know that we're full when we consume these "foods" and drinks.

Carbohydrate, Fat, Protein

Nearly all ultra-processed foods are made up of easily digestible carbohydrates—i.e. highly refined grains and starches and sugars that all **become sugar** (glucose) very quickly in the human body.

It's important to understand why refined carbohydrate negatively affects our health in ways that neither protein nor fat do when it comes to blood sugar, weight, hypertension, and other chronic health problems. There are three key points to keep in mind:

1.) All carbohydrate is **optional** in the human diet provided we eat enough fat and protein

2.) Ultra-processed foods and drinks are **the most damaging types of carbohydrates** because they turn into sugar rapidly in the human body, quickly spiking blood glucose (sugar) and insulin levels. Over time these chronic spikes in blood glucose and insulin levels can cause us to become resistant to our own hormone insulin.

3.) **Ultra-processed foods/drinks and sugar have little to no nutritional value** even if they're "enriched" with synthetic vitamins and minerals added back after they've been fabricated through industrial processes. It's not known if the human body even absorbs these synthetic vitamins and minerals properly—i.e. if they're bioavailable to the human body.

Let's start with the first point above. Unlike protein and fat, which are the two *essential* macronutrients in the human diet, which means mean we must consume them—including fat, **carbohydrate is not an essential macronutrient for humans**.

This means humans can survive and be healthy on protein and fat alone provided we eat adequate amounts of each. (The ketogenic diet does just this by reducing carbs to 5-10% of calories. It is likely humans spent much of our time in ketosis during the millions of years of our evolution.)

The keto diet is just one option on the low-carbohydrate continuum of eating, and you don't necessarily need to follow a strict keto diet in order to transform your health including your blood sugar, weight, blood pressure, cardiovascular health, brain health, and immune system—as long as you're significantly limiting or eliminating **ultra-processed foods and drinks**, as much sugar as you can, **and all forms of fructose** in processed and ultra-processed forms.

Most of us do include carbohydrates in our diet, but it is important to know that they are entirely optional in the human diet, which means you have enormous flexibility and choice when it comes to the carbohydrates you eat.

The best sources of carbohydrate for health are the foods in the first *NOVA* category:

**Vegetables, particularly those that grow above ground because they are much lower
in starch (sugar)**

Beans and legumes

**Unprocessed fruits that are low in sugar such
as berries, tomatoes, avocadoes**

Nuts and seeds in limited portions because they're high in omega-6 fatty acids, which are inflammatory

Genuinely whole grains such as quinoa in limited amounts for reasons we'll discuss

Consuming whole fruit with a lot of sugar such as grapes, bananas, cherries, etc. will make it quite difficult to cut down on sugar consumption in general because their sweetness, which is due to the fructose in them, makes us crave sweetness itself in any form—as well as foods that metabolize quickly into sugar—i.e. ultra-processed foods and drinks.

Therefore, fruits should be considered an *occasional dessert*, not something you consume on a daily basis. The same holds true for "whole grains" because even genuinely whole grains such as quinoa raise blood sugar and insulin levels, which increases hunger and cravings for sweetness. This is how carbohydrate affects the human body.

All grains such as rice, including brown rice, do the same. If you're trying to address cravings for sweet foods, eating a lot of "whole grains" along with fruits is going to make that a lot more difficult to accomplish.

These minimally processed foods are far better than ultra-processed foods and drinks, but if you struggle with cravings for sweet foods, you should limit your consumption of grains and fruits too, especially fruits high in sugar like bananas, grapes, oranges, etc.

All carbohydrate drives hunger and cravings for sweetness, the issue is to what degree. Ultra-processed foods and drinks are going to drive hunger the most quickly and severely. So, focus your meals and snacks on protein, natural fats, and fiber-filled vegetables, nuts and seeds, beans and legumes, which will bring your cravings for sweetness—including sugar—way down.

Since 1980 we've been eating far too much carbohydrate in general and making our meals primarily about carbohydrate, which is a *huge change* from how humans ate for millions of years. This change in the last few decades—i.e. basing our diet on carbohydrate—matters enormously because we evolved as a species eating meat (and seafood) and a lot of fat.

The reason we changed our diets so drastically in 1980 was because that was the first year the U.S. government issued dietary guidelines telling the country, including the nutrition science and medical establishments and institutions, what was healthy to eat and what we should avoid in our diets.

These guidelines were instrumental in making us believe that in order to be healthy we needed to avoid meat and fat, especially natural saturated fat, which meant we had to eat more of something—and that something was carbohydrate, lots of it, and in much more refined, processed, ultra-processed forms.

Food manufacturers took the fat out of foods and replaced it with sugar, hydrogenated oils, trans fats, and high-fructose corn syrup. By getting us to believe that natural sources of fat we'd been eating as a species for millions of years suddenly became dangerous overnight, our standard dietary advice and national dietary guidelines gave the processed food/drink and sugar industries a *huge* boost.

These guidelines were emulated across the globe, which gave the processed food, drink, and sugar industries a huge boost and opened vast new markets and food categories—i.e. the snack. Consequently, the snack food industry absolutely took off as there was now a huge market for refined, processed, ultra-processed foods because they were "low fat." We were told that we needed to snack if we became hungry between meals, something that was highly unusual in human history.

Nutritionists and dieticians routinely told people in the 80's and 90's to eat 6 small meals a day in order to "boost" metabolism and keep up their "energy"—a completely bizarre belief and myth that had absolutely nothing to do with how human metabolism works.

However, as a population we were *suddenly* consuming huge amounts of refined and ultra-processed foods that make humans hungrier, snacking all the time on more of these processed foods, and focusing our meals on carbohydrate.

Doing so began driving our blood sugar and insulin levels up as a population, which resulted in rapid weight gain across the population as well as Type 2 diabetes and hypertension.

This was a massive cultural shift within a very short period of time in relation to human history, and it drastically changed our understanding of what food is, what's nutritionally healthy, how we should eat, and when we should eat. And it all began because of the dogmatic, *un*scientific fear of fat, especially saturated (stable) fat.

The national dietary guidelines first issued in 1980 were not based in science but politics, and they remain *un*scientific to this day, which is deeply tragic and unnecessary. To this day, these guidelines are our national nutrition policy, but they are *not* based in rigorous science. It's a forty-year experiment, without our consent, that has failed miserably and led to our current metabolic health epidemics, including obesity and Type 2 diabetes.

Throughout our evolutionary history as a species, carbohydrate was just a minor adjunct to the human diet, and we consumed natural carbohydrates such as plants and fruits, when we couldn't get animal products such as meat, seafood, and plenty of fat in animal foods.

Carbohydrate was not our priority as a species because it's not nearly as nutritionally dense or satisfying, and it doesn't give us the steady energy of meat, seafood, and natural sources of fat. Carbohydrate also wasn't available most of the time due to geographical location, weather, seasonality, etc., so as a species, we couldn't rely on it, which is why our bodies don't rely on it; they rely on protein and fat.

Archaeological evidence indicates that for millions of years humans didn't eat any carbohydrate. Essentially, humans were forced to start consuming carbohydrates such as plants, nuts and seeds, fruits, etc. because of climate changes and loss of the large, fatty animals, called megafauna, which we hunted, such as mammoths.

We developed weapons and tools for hunting much smaller game such as deer, and we began to supplement our diets by foraging. We can eat natural sources of carbohydrate in plants, nuts and seeds, berries and fruits, but we're not adapted to these as our main diet. We didn't cultivate grains until about 10,000 years ago, so these are incredibly recent foods, and our bodies didn't evolve eating them.

Dairy is also very recent in our history as well. Many people have intolerances/allergies to dairy and grains, particularly to wheat and/or gluten. These are *very* recent foods in our history, which helps to explain why so many people have intolerances and allergies.

Our genes, digestive system, and hormones developed on a diet of meat/seafood and natural sources of fat, **not** carbohydrate. This very sudden shift in our diet in 1980 to high levels of carbohydrate—only the last few decades after millions of years—is not something to which our bodies are accustomed from an evolutionary perspective.

We're designed to eat animal products and a lot of natural fat. It's how our digestive and hormonal systems evolved. We see this most especially in the way a diet high in carbohydrate, especially ultra-processed foods/drinks and sugar, affects our chief hormone, insulin, which is also a very powerful growth factor in the human body.

Fat does not raise insulin, and it was actually used to treat Type 1 diabetes until the invention of exogenous insulin in the early 1920's. It makes complete sense from an evolutionary

—

perspective that fat doesn't raise blood sugar directly or insulin levels because *we ate so much fat* as a species for millions of years.

If fat harmed our blood sugar and insulin levels constantly the way carbohydrate does, we would not have survived as a species. Dietary fat is *not* the enemy when it comes to blood sugar and insulin resistance in the human body.

Natural sources of fat have protective effects on the heart! We are meant to eat fat—in natural sources, including fatty meats and fish. It is uniquely satisfying to humans because we evolved eating it—lots of it.

The same is true of meat. We *evolved* eating meat—*a lot of very fatty meats*—and we ate it raw for millions of years prior to the invention of fire. Our bodies absorb all the vital nutrients in meat and seafood and the fat in them extremely well, which makes perfect sense from an evolutionary perspective.

All foods that contain fat *have all 3 types—monounsaturated, polyunsaturated, and saturated.* This is the natural matrix in which fat occurs in real food.

Our bodies are designed through millions of years of evolution to get different and important nutritional benefits from all 3 types of fat that *always occur together* in natural foods—in different ratios. For example, some types of seafood have a lot more saturated fat than meat does, but we're always told meat is the problem due to the saturated fat, but that fish is always good.

This is mindboggling advice given the actual ratios of saturated fat in some types of fish vis-à-vis meat. When we look at the scientific facts, we often see very widespread misunderstanding in the nutrition science world and medical worlds about what's actually in foods and how they affect the human body.

The notion that we should eat high levels of isolated, industrially fabricated polyunsaturated fat such as toxic "vegetable" oils, which are industrial waste products that don't occur in nature, makes absolutely no sense.

Given our entire evolutionary history and the fact that natural *saturated* fat is also crucial to the body, *especially* to the human brain, which is primarily comprised of fat and cholesterol, we do need to include this type of fat in our diets.

The word "saturated" means that it's *stable* fat at the molecular level: "saturated" is the scientific term that describes these fats, which do not degrade or produce toxic chemicals such as carcinogenic aldehyde when heated as "vegetable" oils do.

We have been taught to *associate* "saturated" with bad and dangerous, but that's not the meaning of "saturated" in terms of its molecular structure: saturated = stable. When we heat saturated fats such as butter or lard or the natural saturated fat in meat and fish, they *don't* degrade quickly into toxic substances that damage the delicate human vascular system.

Fat, especially saturated fat in natural foods, became the enemy in 1980 for reasons that had *nothing to do with science* or how the body works. In 1980 our national dietary guidelines, which were written by politicians (!) and political aides, not scientists, tried to rewrite millions of years of evolutionary history.

During the past forty years, these guidelines have succeeded in getting people to believe that huge amounts of *optional* carbohydrate in the diet is healthy and that both fat, especially saturated fat in natural foods, as well as meat, are dangerous— i.e. the foods we spent millions of years eating.

Our large complex brains evolved *because* we ate these foods, meat and seafood and lots of fat, especially the omega-3 fatty acids in these foods. Our brains aren't made of carbohydrates such as breaded nuggets or pizza or soda; they're about 70% fat!

Cholesterol is *also crucial* to the human brain, and the human brain actually makes and recycles its own cholesterol apart from the body to *ensure* that it has enough. We would not have evolved as a species like this if cholesterol were the enemy.

This is just not how evolution works, but one wouldn't know that given standard dietary and medical advice. Caps on intake of dietary cholesterol have quietly been dropped from our national dietary guidelines, but most in the healthcare professions still believe the entrenched myths and dogma about cholesterol, natural sources of fat, and meat.

Fatty acids are among the most crucial molecules that determine both the brain's integrity and its ability to perform. The essential fatty acids (EFAs), particularly the omega-3 fatty acids we need, cannot be synthesized by the body and must be obtained from dietary
sources. EFAs, as messengers, are also involved in the synthesis and functions of brain neurotransmitters, and in the molecules of the immune system.

These crucial fatty acids are bioavailable to us in animal products because of the way we evolved as a species; plant sources of these crucial fatty acids are far less bioavailable to us for the same reason.

Thus, if you're avoiding *natural* sources of fat in your diet, that's going to have significant implications for your brain as well as cardiovascular health—and stroke risk, particularly if you're a woman.

Just to reiterate—the crucial forms of fat we need as humans come in natural foods that have all 3 types of fat, foods such as meat and seafood and full-fat dairy, *not* toxic vegetable oils like soybean, corn, canola, grape seed, etc.

Nuts and seeds are high in omeg-6 fatty acids, which are inflammatory, so we must be careful to limit consumption of these. During our evolutionary history our diets provided about a 1:1 ratio of omega -6 to omega-3 fatty acids. We do need some omega-6 fatty acids in our diet.

However, our diets are now a 20:1 ratio of inflammatory omega -6 fatty acids to omega-3's. They're completely out of balance—and toxic, highly inflammatory "vegetable" oils are the main culprits.

Our national dietary guidelines have changed remarkably little in 40 years—the same years in which obesity, Type 2 diabetes, hypertension, cholesterol problems, NAFLD began to skyrocket—all driven by a diet high in carbohydrate and especially ultra-processed foods and drinks and sugar.

Cardiovascular disease is getting worse, not better, despite all the advances in medical care. People no longer smoke as they did from the 1950's to the 1980's, which was a major cause of heart disease. Cardiovascular disease rates should have dropped significantly as a result. They haven't.

Ultra-processed foods, drinks, sugar, and toxic vegetable oils since 1980 are the primary causes of the harm to our hearts and cardiovascular systems—via inflammation and insulin resistance due to diet.

Again, we don't absorb vitamins and other nutrients, such as important fatty acids, from plant sources nearly as well as we do from animal sources. This isn't political; it's due to our evolutionary history. This is the reason vegetarians and vegans *must supplement carefully* in order to get a nutritionally complete diet.

We *can* eat carbohydrate, but it raises blood sugar and insulin levels in ways that neither protein or fat do—and it's these spikes blood sugar and insulin over time that lead to our chronic metabolic diseases and conditions.

Since 1980 we have been consuming *enormous* amounts of carbohydrate, most especially in ultra-processed foods and drinks as well as sugar, causing *rapid* increases in health problems including prediabetes and Type 2diabetes, hypertension, obesity, cardiovascular disease, cholesterol problems, and dementia.

The brain is exquisitely sensitive to sugar and foods that metabolize quickly into sugar such as ultra-processed foods and drinks. Insulin can't cross the blood-brain barrier, **so blood sugar stays high in the brain**—killing brain cells.

Ultra-processed foods and drinks, particularly sugar in all its forms, mean that the brain ends up swimming in glucose (sugar) that it can't use because insulin can't get in to usher it into cells.

Our bodies work in ways that are truly ancient—millions of years old—which is why our carbohydrate-centered, ultra-processed diet since 1980 is so deeply incompatible with human health, our genes, our hormonal system, our brains, our hearts, our livers, our immune system—and every other aspect of our bodies and how they work.

Our bodies did not evolve over the vast sweep of time (millions of years) to consume ultra-processed foods and sugar that are essentially toxic to us as a species. They don't kill us quickly like toxic plants or fungi; instead ultra-processed substances kill us slowly via metabolic diseases and conditions, particularly those driven by insulin resistance, which we'll discuss.

The longer we eat a carbohydrate-centered diet that's especially high in ultra-processed foods and drinks, the worse our chronic metabolic diseases and conditions become as individuals and as a population.

We see this in very stark ways in all the health data that shows dramatic increases in Type 2 diabetes, obesity, NAFLD, hypertension, dementia, cardiovascular disease, and other diet-driven chronic health problems—all since 1980 when we started being advised to eat in ways that had no foundation at all in rigorous science.

The ultra-processed food industry has been taking every possible advantage of these dietary guidelines ever since, which is why the industry now dominates our food supply—and our diets.

It is not a coincidence that our metabolic health has declined precipitously as a population since 1980, across all age groups, including among teenagers, children, and even babies who now get "adult" diseases such as Type 2 diabetes and obesity.

Babies get these diseases now because all the same ultra-processed ingredients and toxins, especially sugar and fructose, are widely used in foods and drinks made for babies and children. These "foods" are ubiquitous in school lunches—because they comply with our national dietary guidelines.

This tells us something is very, very wrong with our food supply *and* our dietary advice. If our national dietary guidelines were scientific and proven to maintain good health, our health wouldn't be getting so much worse. All the data show we are following these guidelines, so it's not about lack of compliance.

"Compliance" or adherence is the measurement used to determine the "success" of our national dietary guidelines—*not* whether these guidelines actually maintain or improve health. Essentially, the dietary guidelines are "successful" when people comply with them and all the standard dietary advice that flows from them.

Whether this advice actually works regarding human health is not the standard by which these guidelines are, or have ever been, measured. That's very dangerous, and no other field of science works this way.

The guidelines are a key part of the problem, and they always have been a driver of poor health in the U.S. This is because these guidelines are responsible for shifting our diets away from protein and fat, which are essential to humans, and emphasizing carbohydrate, which is optional.

As national nutrition policy, these guidelines are responsible for our diets and food supply becoming flooding with ultra-processed, toxic, and addictive substances and for determining the standard dietary advice we can be given as well as the foods millions of people are allowed to eat in a wide range of institutions and through programs such as school lunches and supplemental feeding programs for the most economically vulnerable citizens.

The guidelines made all of this feasible by changing our beliefs, habits, and assumptions about the "dangers" of meat and natural fat and championing the "benefits" of carbohydrate and refined carbohydrate in particular—and doing so as *national policy*.

Despite knowing the diet-driven diseases that now dominate our national healthcare system, our national dietary guidelines continue to tell Americans to eat like this.

These guidelines resulted in massive changes throughout out entire food supply and to the dramatic rise in the availability and consumption of ultra-processed foods and drinks as well as sugar. Animals were suddenly bred to be much leaner, so we were no longer getting the essential natural fat, including saturated fat, which the human body must have.

Consequently, all the metabolic diseases and conditions we're experiencing across all age groups are the direct result of **carbohydrate toxicity**, which happens when we're eating far more carbohydrate than our bodies can metabolize properly. This happens especially quickly when we're consuming ultra-processed foods and drinks, particularly sugar in its 260+ forms.

When we eat ultra-processed foods/drinks and sugar in any form, *we can develop carbohydrate toxicity very quickly*—leading to **insulin resistance**, which is at the root of most of our chronic health problems—a condition we'll discuss in the next section.

All the excess glucose (sugar) from a diet high in carbohydrate, especially ultra-processed foods and drinks and sugar in all forms, also ends up getting stored as **fat** in our organs and in our fat cells—because the human body can't store carbohydrate directly.

Our bodies convert it into glucose, and if we're not burning it up through *a lot of ongoing physical activity throughout our waking hours*, the hormone insulin prompts our bodies to store that glucose as fat.

This is millions of years of evolutionary adaptations at work, and this evolutionary reality won't change despite the nonsense we're constant told by ultra-processed "food" and drink makers such as "a calorie is a calorie," which is not true.

What matters is *what our bodies do* with the protein, fat, and carbohydrates we consume, and that depends entirely on what kind of protein, fat, and carbohydrates we're consuming.

A calorie is *not* a calorie. That's complete nonsense in terms of human metabolism and biochemistry.

Ultra-processed food and drink manufacturers *want you* to believe this utter nonsense about calories because "calories" *make it seem like we're choosing* how our bodies metabolize carbohydrate, fat and protein via how many "calories" we consume or burn.

We don't "choose" how to metabolize foods/drinks, and we don't choose how these foods and drinks affect our hormones such as leptin and insulin.

What matters is *how* our bodies metabolize protein, carbohydrate, and fat very differently, which has profound implications for our health.

The calories in ultra-processed foods/drinks *are not the same* as the calories in whole foods such as cheddar cheese or meat or vegetables, etc. in terms of what our bodies *do* with these foods.

Calories tell us *absolutely nothing* about how our bodies metabolize these foods or how foods/drinks directly affect our hormones such as insulin (fat storage hormone) or leptin (appetite/satiety hormone).

Natural cheddar cheese or meat has a lot more calories, but they're not going to spike blood sugar or insulin levels, and they're going to give you essential protein and fat and vitamins and minerals that your body *needs*.

They're going to leave you full and satisfied because the protein and the fat in them are the things *the human body must have* for everything the body does every day including maintaining bone density and all our cells, maintaining the immune system, ensuring the brain's many complex functions, etc.

The body *uses protein and fat for the vast majority of our needs* on a daily basis—i.e. all the things our bodies do without our input. This is protein and fat, not carbohydrates, *doing all this work every day*.

This is how we evolved as a species, which is why protein and fat are essential to our health to this day and why carbohydrate, which was not part of our diet for millions of years, is not essential.

Our bodies turn protein into glucose at a lower rate, so we're never going to run out of "energy" as we're so often told by dietary authorities when they advise us to center our diets on carbohydrate for the "energy"—high levels of sugar.

Ultra-processed foods/drinks may have far fewer "calories," but they're going to spike your blood sugar and insulin levels causing fat storage, cravings, and increased hunger, provide next to no bioavailable nutrients. The fats in them are usually the inflammatory, toxic "vegetable" oils that harm our health.

These ultra-processed substances are not going to give you the protein and natural sources of fat your body must have in order to function and survive and be healthy.

Because they don't give us what our bodies need and must have, we end up craving more and more of these substances, and we get hungrier—because our bodies *are starving*—they're getting nothing they need and must have for survival from these "foods." This is why obesity and serious nutritional deficiencies so often happen together.

Summary: all carbohydrate is optional in the human diet provided we're eating enough of the two things that are absolutely essential in the human diet: **fat and protein**. This means we can and should be very selective about the carbohydrates we choose to eat, and how much carbohydrate we eat.

All carbohydrate is addictive *to some degree* to the human species; it raises blood sugar and insulin levels, and drives hunger. Sugar is the carbohydrate that raises blood sugar and insulin the most, is the most addictive, and increases hunger the most. It also has **no** nutritional value. *Sugar is not a food; it's a toxin.*

Thus, we should focus on whole and natural carbohydrates as much as possible, including low-starch vegetables, low-sugar fruits such as berries and tomatoes, limited nuts and seeds, and very limited whole grains such as quinoa that we make at home.

We should focus on eating whole and nature foods, including foods that have natural fat (all 3 kinds) such as meat, seafood, full-fat, unsweetened dairy, butter, cheese, etc. and not obsess about "calories," because *the body has no receptors for "calories;"* this means the body doesn't recognize or metabolize what we eat and drink according to "calories."

The human body understands and metabolizes *protein and fat* for nearly all its needs, and it recognizes carbohydrate that it converts into glucose (sugar) for immediate energy—i.e. physical exertion. Too much carbohydrate leads to carbohydrate toxicity because, as a species, we didn't evolve eating carbohydrate—let alone toxic ultra-processed foods and drinks.

We can eat carbohydrate in general, but it affects us very differently in terms of our health—most especially via the hormones insulin and leptin. Ultra-processed foods and drinks are, essentially, alien substances to the human body.

We won't die immediately when we consume them as we will with poisonous plants and fungi, but these substances cause serious havoc with our organs, cells, and hormones and lead to chronic metabolic health problems, primarily by causing insulin resistance.

Finally, remember that our cells, organ, genes, and hormonal system can't do arithmetic—i.e. add or subtract "calories." The body metabolizes carbohydrate, fat, and protein; calories are just a way of *talking* about foods/drinks that comes from the nineteenth century (!)

"Calories" have nothing to do with what our bodies are actually *doing* with what we eat and drink, which is what matters.

Insulin Resistance and Ultra-Processed Foods/Drinks and Sugar

Nearly all ultra-processed foods are carbohydrates, and all carbohydrate raises blood sugar (glucose) and prompts insulin secretion. All carbohydrate is also optional if you're eating enough protein *and* fat.

Protein also increases blood glucose, but it's a very distant second behind carbohydrate. Our liver also makes glucose, so our brains are never without the glucose they need. Our liver does this every morning so we have enough energy to wake up! This process is called gluconeogenesis.

Dietary fat does not raise blood sugar directly or insulin levels. Fat does not make us fat. Chronically elevated insulin in the blood from a diet high in easily digestible carbohydrates and sugar, ultra-processed foods and drinks, causes our bodies to go into fat storage overdrive via the hormone insulin.

Let's look at how this process works. When we consume any food/drink, our blood sugar goes up; when this happens, our pancreas gland automatically secretes insulin in order to dispose of that glucose (sugar) in our blood—either by ushering it into our cells to be used for energy or to be stored as fat.

Insulin does one or the other, not both at the same time, which is very important to remember.

If we're not using all the glucose (sugar) from the foods/drinks we consume for our actual energy needs such as physical activity throughout the day, we're going to store it as fat in our organs and fat cells—i.e. we're going to gain weight.

When we're eating a diet focused on carbohydrates that turn quickly into sugar, i.e. ultra-processed foods/drinks and sugar, we're far more likely to gain weight quickly and have considerable difficulty in taking it off.

Chronically high spikes in blood sugar over time from a diet high in carbohydrate, especially ultra-processed foods and sugar, *means* chronically high spikes in insulin too. Over time these constant spikes in the hormone insulin cause our cells to start ignoring insulin, which means insulin has considerable difficulty ushering glucose into the cells the be used for energy.

When this happens, our blood sugar starts to stay high all the time, leading to prediabetes and then Type 2 diabetes. This process in which our own cells ignore our own powerful hormone insulin is called **insulin resistance**.

Unlike protein and fat, which are the two essential macronutrients in our diet, carbohydrate is the optional macronutrient in our diet that *single-handedly* causes insulin resistance, weight gain & obesity, prediabetes and Type 2 diabetes, high blood pressure, and cholesterol problems (high triglycerides). This happens most often via the process of insulin resistance.

In turn, these diet-driven diseases and conditions drive the development of cardiovascular disease, nonalcoholic fatty liver disease (NAFLD), and dementia. Essentially cardiovascular disease is diabetes of the heart and dementia is diabetes of the brain.

All of these chronic metabolic diseases and conditions driven by insulin resistance now affect **88% of American adults.** [5]At the root of insulin resistance, which is a dietary condition in the vast majority of cases, are easily digestible carbohydrates—i.e. ultra-processed foods and drinks and far too much sugar and fructose.

Thus, it's ultra-processed foods and drinks, not meat or healthy dietary fat in natural foods such as butter, cheese, cream etc. that are doing so much damage to all areas of our health, including our weight.

The reason for this is because **insulin is also our fat storage hormone**, and when we eat these ultra-processed foods and drinks that constantly spike our blood sugar and insulin, we're keeping our fat storage hormone insulin chronically elevated. When we do this, we're constantly *telling* our bodies to store fat and not to release it.

When we store fat in our organs such as the liver (as well as the pancreas gland which secretes insulin), we damage these organs and glands—most especially the liver, which causes the liver to become insulin resistant over time.

When the liver becomes fatty, it's called nonalcoholic fatty liver disease (NAFLD); as the liver becomes increasingly insulin resistant this drives insulin resistance globally throughout the body.

---

[5] Joana Araújo, Jianwen Cai, and June Stevens. Prevalence of Optimal Metabolic Health in American Adults: National Health and Nutrition Examination Survey 2009–2016. *Metabolic Syndrome and Related Disorders*. Feb 2019.46-52. http://doi.org/10.1089/met.2018.0105

Finally, when our insulin levels stay high all the time, which is called **hyperinsulinemia**, our fat cells can't release fatty acids; the reason for this is that high levels of insulin work like a hormonal lock preventing the release of fatty acids (i.e. fat.)

It's ultra-processed foods and drinks that drive food cravings, spike blood sugar and insulin responses the most, cause our bodies to store fat and prevent release of fat. Sugar in particular is highly inflammatory and suppresses the immune system, leaving us more vulnerable to a range of infections as well as infectious diseases.

Ultra-processed foods/drinks, especially sugar and high levels of fructose in processed foods and drinks, are driving all the chronic metabolic diseases and conditions that are now responsible for **75% of all healthcare costs**, and the situation is getting worse each year across the globe as billions of people consume greater quantities of ultra-processed foods and drinks.

Making the decision to eliminate or significantly limit your consumption of ultra-processed foods and drinks as well as sugar is the single most important thing you can do for *every* aspect of your health, now and for the future.

Plant-based Ultra-Processed Foods

Much of the "plant-based" movement is actually an extremely well-funded and orchestrated campaign to keep selling us the same addictive substances made to look like new "foods."

These toxic substances actually harm the planet given how they're produced—from all the pesticides used to grow the cheap grains, starches, and sugars from which these "foods" are made to the deforestation to grow these monocrops, to the wildlife that is destroyed through agricultural harvesting methods including huge combine harvesters.

"Plant-based" is essentially the newest deflection technique for keeping us addicted to these ultra-processed foods and drinks while getting us think we're doing something positive for the environment by consuming them.

All the money goes into getting us hooked on these "foods," manipulating perceptions about convenience and fulfillment (physical, emotional, etc.), and now using the climate crisis to convince us that consuming these "plant-based," highly refined grains, sugars, starches, and toxic oils will help the planet, which has no basis in science or fact.

This is not to say the meat and dairy industries don't need serious reform; they do. However, animals are *crucial* to regenerative agriculture—i.e. to nourishing and replenishing vital topsoil by walking on it, leaving their rich dung, etc.

We're feeding cows corn and other substances *they can't digest properly*, which is why they produce methane. Cows *are not* the problem; factory farming and what we feed the cows are the problem. It's what we are doing to the cows that's causing the problem in terms of climate issues.

Much land is not suitable to agricultural farming of monocrops, but it is suitable for grazing animals that replenish the soil and provide food products that are highly nutritious and bioavailable to humans.

This "plant-based" rhetoric has quickly become a cornerstone of the ultra-and processed food giants. Convincing people they should eat ultra-processed foods to save the planet is *designed* to divert attention and focus from the industries that have and continue to cause exponentially more harm to the planet in terms of global warming than animal products do. It's a diversionary tactic, and it works.

The "plant-based" corporations and entities—primarily junk food companies—are quickly being joined by the fast food companies that are now rushing to offer customers the cheapest most addictive and toxic ingredients wrapped in "eco" consciousness.

The reality is that these cheap carbohydrates (grains, sugars, starches, sugars, chemicals, and "vegetable" oils) are far cheaper for them than meat, and the profits are much higher. Saving the planet has *nothing* to do with it; it's all about the money.

If you're vegan or vegetarian, these "plant-based" substances are not about "plant-based" eating; they're about profits and the patents on these "foods" and the techniques and equipment used to make them that are incredibly lucrative. It's about controlling sectors of the food supply, lucrative patents, and making trillions.

If you are vegetarian or vegan, *please*—eat a diet of whole, unprocessed plants, nuts and seeds, beans and legumes, good sources of natural fats like olives, olive oil, coconut and coconut oil and avocadoes, and consume limited whole fruit low in sugar and limited *genuinely whole* grains.

Do not fall for the toxic, "plant-based," ultra-processed foods and drinks; they're also insanely expensive for a toxic pile of sludge with food coloring, flavorings, and all the other junk.

Their Nutrition Facts labels are just as misleading as these labels are on other products, and their ingredient lists are equally horrifying as anything else that's ultra-processed. This "plant-based" stuff is not food no matter what the big investors and Wall St. tell us.

It's all about very profitable new food markets for the same cheap, toxic ingredients that harm our soil and environment through massive use of pesticides, causing dead zones in our oceans and harming marine life, as well as harmful harvesting techniques. It's about owning parts of our food supply itself through patents.

One can't patent plants or animals or other products of nature, but these investors are *very* busy putting patents on entire food categories such as fake meats. This will affect our food supply in ways that may seem inconceivable to us now, but it will happen.

This is how control of the food supply works. We've *already* seen this—i.e. in the 1980's with the low-fat, high-carb, toxic and refined "foods" flooding our stores, changing our agricultural practices, our meats and dairy (which all became low fat), our food supply, and our health.

For example, an airline billionaire gets to tell us we need to eat toxic, highly refined and ultra-processed junk made to look like meat in order to combat climate change—after making billions through decades of harming the global climate—when the science was well known. It's about the money, the patents, the lucrative markets, and owning entire sectors the food supply.

Eat real plants, grains, vegetables, beans/legumes, nuts and seeds, limited low-sugar fruits, plenty of natural fats—and don't go within a country mile of this toxic "plant-based" nonsense

---

wrapped in lectures from those who have already done substantial damage to the planet—and made enormous profits doing it.

The point here is that the ultra-processed food and drink industries, including fast food, are intentionally manipulating our deep concern and anxiety about climate change to sell us *more* ultra-processed foods and drinks that actually cause environmental devastation in myriad ways—and continue to make us very sick.

A very sick human population globally due to a diet high in ultra-processed foods/drinks and sugar is also not good for the planet and its limited resources.

If one is vegetarian or vegan, one should eat whole foods using the *NOVA* system—not toxic "plant-based" ultra-processed foods and drinks that do such damage to our bodies, minds, and spirits—*and* to the planet.

Ultra-Processed Foods/Drinks and the Dangers of Fructose

The human body uses glucose (sugar) for many purposes. Our bodies turn the foods and drinks we consume into glucose at different rates; the more natural and unprocessed the food the *more slowly it becomes glucose.* Protein does become glucose, but at a much slower rate than carbohydrate.

Fat does not raise blood sugar directly or raise insulin levels, and in fact fat was used as the treatment for Type 1 diabetes prior to the invention of exogenous insulin in the early 1920's.

Unlike glucose, only the liver can process **fructose**, which is the molecule in table sugar that makes it sweet. Table sugar is 50% sucrose and 50% fructose. Sodas and other liquids with fructose *are especially damaging to the liver because they're in liquid form,* i.e. there's no fiber to slow the rate at which the concentrated fructose hits the liver.

Fructose slams the liver very hard becoming liver fat and making the liver insulin resistant. When the liver is insulin resistant, it drives insulin resistance throughout the human body.

Juices also contain a high amount of sugar and fructose, which is why they're also a serious problem for the liver. The sugar in them spikes blood sugar and insulin levels quickly, and the fructose can only be handled by the liver, which means the burden of dealing with fructose falls entirely on this vital organ.

The fructose in sodas is even worse for the liver. Whole fruit contains fructose and sugar, but the fiber in it slows the rate at which these are metabolized.

So, *sodas and drinks with fructose in any form and sugar are absolutely the worst things to consume.* Juices are also a problem because of the sugar and fructose in them—and many juices have added sugar as well.

Whole, natural fruits with all the fiber intact are the least damaging to blood sugar and insulin levels and to the liver, but they still have high levels of sugar, so they can't and shouldn't be considered something we eat daily as part of a healthy diet.

In the middle of the last century, high-fructose corn syrup and huge amounts of sugar entered our diets in unprecedented ways. Our consumption of sugar went up significantly as did our consumption of ultra-processed foods that all become sugar (glucose) very quickly in the body.

These foods flooded the food supply throughout the U.S. as well as other countries. When one looks at the data over time, the enormous rise in chronic metabolic diseases and conditions such as Type 2 diabetes, obesity / weight gain, hypertension, cardiovascular diseases, and cholesterol problems *tracks in lockstep with these dietary changes.*

These dietary changes are substantially increased consumption of ultra-processed foods, far more sugar, trans fats (now removed from the food supply) and a lot more fructose in processed foods and drinks.

Metabolic Syndrome

Cutting consumption of ultra-processed foods and drinks (especially sugar and fructose) will absolutely make a huge difference regarding a cluster of health problems that was originally known as "syndrome x," the term coined by the pioneering endocrinologist, Gerald Reaven.

It's a cluster of interrelated problems we now call **metabolic syndrome**: *high blood pressure, high blood sugar, excess body fat around the waist, and abnormal HDL cholesterol/triglyceride levels.* Protein and fat, the other two macronutrients in our diets in addition to carbohydrate, **do not drive metabolic syndrome**.

As we've discussed, you can live perfectly well without consuming any carbs at all provided you're eating adequate protein and fat. This is essentially the keto diet, which means your liver converts fat (from your diet and the fat on your body) into ketones, which the body uses instead of glucose for energy. The liver continues to make the glucose (sugar) your brain must have through the process of gluconeogenesis.

If you have Metabolic Syndrome, or NAFLD, know that limiting or eliminating ultra-processed foods and drinks is *the most important thing you can do* to prevent these conditions from worsening. For many people, it's also possible to reverse one or both of these conditions—and diet is the only way to do so.

The same is true of prediabetes and in many cases, Type 2 diabetes. Diet is the tool that works; there is no drug that affects the cellular pathways of insulin resistance, which is what causes high blood sugar and so many other chronic health problems.

Therefore, if you have high blood sugar, limiting/eliminating ultra-processed foods and drinks as well as sugar in all its forms will make *the biggest difference* in reversing the insulin resistance driving these conditions.

Your body can become far more insulin sensitive again, and removing all the foods that rapidly metabolize into sugar—ultra-process foods and drinks—as well as sugar itself are the only ways to do this.

Drugs don't reverse insulin resistance, which is a dietary condition; changing your diet is how your reverse this condition—now and for the future.

Along the way, you'll also notice that your blood pressure improves; the reason for this is that in the vast majority of cases, sugar is the culprit behind hypertension. Too much salt in the diet will worsen it—but salt doesn't cause high blood pressure.

Sugar and foods that rapidly metabolize into sugar (and therefore cause weight gain too) are the causal problem.

Finally, if you have high triglycerides, you'll soon notice that a diet low in ultra-processed foods/drinks and sugar brings your triglycerides down. (Triglycerides are a type of fat that's dangerous for our cardiovascular health, among other things.)

Triglycerides are a direct measurement of the carbohydrate in our diet, so in focusing your diet on whole, natural foods, low-sugar fruits such as berries, avocadoes, and tomatoes, as well as low-starch vegetables, nuts and seeds, beans and legume, meat and fish, and natural sources of fat, you'll find that your triglycerides look much better on your tests results.

Finally, if you have low HDL, the "good" cholesterol, there are only two things that can improve it: months of consistent exercise and saturated fat in the diet. Yes, you read that correctly! Saturated fat is the **only food** known to improve HDL cholesterol.

So when you're enjoying some butter, cheese, full-fat dairy, meat and seafood with saturated fat, you're improving your "good" cholesterol too. ("Vegetable" or "plant-based" industrial oils do not provide this benefit.)

Ultra-Processed Foods and Sugar Deliberately Target and Exploit Our Evolutionary Vulnerabilities as Humans, Including Inherent Cravings for Sweet Food and Susceptibility to Weight Gain as a Species

Given that sugar and all ultra-processed foods and drinks are inherently addictive, we're all vulnerable when it comes to these substances. These "foods" are addictive because they exploit *our shared evolutionary drives and cravings for sweet foods and foods that metabolize rapidly into sugar and spike our blood glucose*, which is what all refined and processed grains, starches, and sugar do.

Savory ultra-processed foods such as potato chips and French fries become sugar (glucose) in your body very quickly—spiking blood sugar and insulin levels.

Even if the ultra-processed food doesn't contain "added" sugar, it all becomes sugar very quickly inside our bodies. This is one of the many reasons Nutrition Fact labels that tell us how much "added" sugar is in something are completely misleading.

These labels do not tell us what the *human body does* with these foods—i.e. how it metabolizes them, beginning with when foods/drinks hit the tongue, which then sends signals to our brains.

The brain then sends the message to our pancreas gland to secrete insulin—and if the taste is sweet on our tongues—to secrete a lot of insulin because something very sweet has just entered the body.

Our bodies get the signals that a large amount of insulin will be needed to dispose of all the glucose that is about to enter our blood from what we've just consumed that's so sweet in taste.

This is why artificial sweeteners and sugar alternatives are such a problem; our bodies *understand* them as very sweet and to release a lot of insulin—even though there's no "calories" in them and no glucose entering our blood from them. They don't raise blood sugar necessarily—but they do spike insulin response.

Remember, chronic spikes in insulin cause insulin resistance and hyperinsulinemia over time, which drive pre-diabetes, Type 2 diabetes, and weight gain—because insulin is also our fat storage hormone that tells our bodies to store fat.

Why are we vulnerable to ultra-processed foods/drinks and sugar that spike blood glucose and insulin levels? *It's due to our evolutionary history as a species*, not lack of willpower, or "calories." When we consume carbohydrate, sources of which are rare in nature, our blood sugar and insulin levels go up—far more so than when we eat protein, *and fat does not raise blood sugar directly or raise insulin levels.*

When we eat ultra-processed foods/drinks and sugar, we spike our blood glucose (sugar) and therefore insulin levels the most. Our bodies are made to use this sugar (glucose) for immediate energy, which we're not doing as a population. Consuming ultra-processed foods/drinks and sugar means we have chronic, high spikes in blood sugar, which we're immediately using (burning) for our energy needs.

All this excess glucose (sugar) has to go somewhere, and it does: insulin tells our bodies to store it as fat because that's one of the key jobs inulin has in the human body.

Why do our bodies do this with excess glucose (sugar) from our diet? It's so that we'll have a source of energy for later when there is no food: the fat we store in our bodies—including in our organs. The human body is *made to preserve, not lose, fat* because fat meant survival for millions of years of our evolutionary history.

—

Our bodies still work exactly this way; our bodies *still prioritize* gaining and maintaining weight, not losing it.

For millions of years, we *often* had to go for days or even weeks without a source of food due to weather, illness, injury, lack of animals to hunt, climate factors, etc. We could *only* survive if we had fat on our bodies to burn for energy, which is exactly what humans did all the time for millions of years.

This is how the keto or ketogenic diet works; it lowers carbohydrate intake low enough that our bodies turn to our stored energy, fat, turning into ketones, which the entire body, including the brain, uses for energy instead of glucose/sugar.

This is why losing weight and keeping it off is so very difficult; doing so goes against our entire evolutionary history as a species. Our bodies are adapted to gain weight and not lose it— that's evolution at work. *We* don't want this to happen, but that's how the human body works because fat meant survival in terms of the millions of years of our evolutionary history.

Thus, when we consume ultra-processed foods/drinks and sugar, we're telling our bodies to store all the excess glucose (sugar) into which these substances metabolize *rapidly*—as fat.

This is also a key reason these "foods" and sugar are also so attractive to us—at an evolutionary level—because they rapidly dump a lot of sugar (glucose) into our blood, sugar that excites our brain cells before killing them—i.e. sugar rush—and then we store the vast majority of this glucose as fat for later.

Ultra-processed foods and drinks and refined sugar don't exist in nature, which is very important to remember because our bodies evolved, including 99% of our genes and our hormonal system, in response to the foods we ate for millions of years, which were almost exclusively animal products (meat and fat), which don't spike blood sugar and insulin levels the way carbohydrate does.

Our bodies are also adapted, over millions of years, to eat carbohydrate, protein, and fat *in whole foods*—i.e. a food in its natural matrix. Our bodies are not adapted to consume isolated, refined, protein, fat, carbs, sugar, etc. The entire food is what is legible, so to speak, to the human body—not isolated components that are refined from foods.

Ultra-processed foods/drinks and sugar hit our tongues, which send messages to our brains as all foods/drinks do; the message in this case is that we're consuming something *highly unusual* (not found in nature) that will give us a *unique chance* spike blood sugar (glucose) so we can store a lot of fat via the automatic insulin spike.

To the human body, sweet foods/drinks and foods that rapidly raise blood sugar mean a chance to store energy for later (fat). This is how our bodies understand ultra-processed foods/drinks and sugar at the hormonal level.

To the human body, ultra-processed foods, drinks, and sugar are essentially an *anomaly*—they're not normal because they are not the norm in nature—and our bodies know this beginning with when these substances hit our tongues. Our hormones know ultra-processed foods/drinks and refined sugars under 260 names are not normal—i.e. the norm in nature, and our bodies respond to these highly unusual substances accordingly.

Ultra-processed foods/drinks and sugar in 260+ forms are norm in our current food environments, *but to the human body, these substances are incredibly unusual because we didn't evolve consuming them.* Our bodies interpret these substances, which don't exist in nature, as a *highly unique way* to gain more fat, which evolution drives our bodies to do.

Again, gaining and maintain our highest weight is not what we want, but it's what our bodies do because they're designed through millions of years to do this.

We are not conscious of this when we buy ultra-processed foods and drinks, but these *evolutionary* drives are incredibly strong in us, which is why they're so difficult to resist.

The companies that make ultra-processed foods and drinks and put sugar in everything know this evolutionary history all too well; they know that it's incredibly difficult to resist the inherent appeal of these highly unusual substances not found in nature because *we're wired to pay attention* to anything that enables us to raise blood sugar rapidly and store all this excess glucose as fat to be used later for energy when there is no food.

That's how we're made as a species, and these companies deliberately exploit this evolutionary history and reality.

The appeal of ultra-processed foods/drinks isn't a failure of personal willpower; it's how these companies use evolutionary forces that are millions of years old against us in order to addict us and keep us eating/drinking these toxic substances.

Edible carbohydrates are rare in nature as the vast majority of plants are toxic to us, and we only began cultivating grains 10,000 years ago when the majority of our genes as a species were already established in response to eating meat and fat—animals—not carbohydrate. Sources of sugar like seasonal fruits and honey very rare in nature.

During our evolutionary history if we found a source of food (carbohydrate) that spiked blood sugar a lot, such as honey or seasonal fruits such as berries or apples, we would eat a lot of it—if we got to it before other animals that also eat these foods.

We'd become *temporarily* insulin resistant in response—i.e. our bodies would pump out a lot of insulin in response to eating those berries or apples or honey. This temporary insulin resistance enabled us to store fat because insulin is our fat storage hormone.

This is exactly how our bodies are *designed* to work—and it's based on the fact that carbohydrate is rare in nature, and we didn't consume much of it, and we went for long periods without consuming any of it.

Evolutionary adaptations ensured that our bodies are not dependent on rare sources of carbohydrate in nature. Second, evolutionary adaptations ensured that our bodies could maximize the rare carbohydrates we did consume by turning it glucose quickly and storing it as fat to burn later.

Now we're eating a diet high in ultra-processed foods/drinks and sugar *that work in exactly the same ways*—they spike blood sugar and make us insulin resistant so we'll store all that excess glucose as fat—but the difference is we're eating highly refined and processed carbohydrates all the time.

We're no longer temporarily insulin resistant in response to eating a bunch of honey or berries that we might happen to find once in a while. We're chronically insulin resistant as a population in response to a diet centered on carbohydrate and especially from eating ultra-processed foods/drinks and sugar.

Finally, we're not burning our stored fat for energy as we did throughout our evolutionary history as a species, so we're chronically building our fat stores.

Summary: the human body is adapted to becoming temporarily insulin resistant in response to rare sources of carbohydrate in nature such as honey, seasonal fruits, plants, tubers, etc.

Agriculture and grain cultivation are incredibly recent inventions in our evolutionary history, and for millions of years during which our genes, digestive and hormonal systems evolved, we ate primarily animal products: meat and a lot of fat in those meats.

We can eat carbohydrate, but our bodies respond to it in ways that differ from protein and fat. Carbohydrate raises blood sugar and insulin levels in ways that protein and fat do not.

When our glucose (sugar) goes up more in response to carbohydrate, our bodies have to either burn this excess glucose for our immediate energy needs or store it as fat because humans can't store carbohydrate directly.

The hormone insulin does both jobs—facilitates getting glucose into the cells for energy or into cells to be stored as fat, but it can't do these jobs at the same time.

From an evolutionary perspective, this process makes complete sense because high blood sugar in response to consuming carbohydrate = high insulin secretion = storing more fat, which meant survival when we didn't have food, which happened throughout our history as a species.

Ultra-processed foods/drinks and sugar are completely anomalous because they are not found in nature, so our bodies respond to them in ways that differ significantly from our responses to natural foods that always exist within a larger matrix of protein, *all 3 types of fat* (mono-poly-and saturated fat) in any natural food that contains fat, fiber, water, macronutrients and micronutrients.

Our bodies are designed to metabolize a food within its entire natural matrix, not isolated ingredients from which the entire matrix (complexity) of a food has been removed and stripped out. This means all the refined flours, starches, and sugars in ultra-processed foods speed through our bodies to become sugar very quickly.

Ultra-processed foods/drinks and sugar are comprised of a very few isolated ingredients stripped of all complexity (natural matrix.) These substances are designed and manufactured to *trigger* the process of spiking blood sugar significantly, which immediately affects the pleasure responses in the brain, so we'll *seek out* more sweet foods and ultra-processed foods/drinks that raise blood sugar quickly affecting the brain.

Ultra-processed foods/drinks rapidly start to metabolize into sugar *from the moment they hit our tongues* sending the signal to our brains that our blood sugar is going to go up rapidly; our brains then send the signal to the pancreas to secrete a lot of insulin.

These foods become sugar *on our tongues* because they have been stripped of their natural matrix in which the fiber, water, protein, all 3 types of fat, etc. slow the rate at which we metabolize a whole and natural food into glucose.

From an evolutionary perspective, high blood sugar = high insulin secretion = storing more fat. Essentially, our bodies understand ultra-processed foods, drinks, and sugar as highly unusual opportunities to become insulin resistant and store fat. Our bodies understand fat storage as a survival advantage because it was for millions of years.

Thus, we seek out these ultra-processed foods, drinks and sugar because we're driven to prioritize any food, especially rare carbohydrates, that let us build up our energy stores—our fat— to be used when we couldn't find food later.

This isn't a conscious process; it's instinctual, and the companies that make ultra-processed foods and drinks know it's *extremely* difficult to go against instincts that are hardwired into a species, humans include.

These evolutionary metabolic processes have not changed. What has changed so significantly is the food—especially the ways in which our diets and stores became flooded with ultra-processed foods, drinks, and sugar.

These are substances that don't exist in nature; but now they dominate our food environments. This isn't about nostalgia for some mythic evolutionary past.

At metabolic, biochemical, hormonal levels, our bodies work properly when we consume the foods we ate for millions of years. It's the way we've evolved, and our bodies are not going to change to accommodate the junk food industry that dominates the culture. We'll just keep getting sicker.

When we eat ultra-processed foods/drinks and sugar, our bodies turn these highly unusual substances into something our bodies can use—fat for energy.

However, as a population, we're not using our fat this way as we did for millions of years because we no longer have to hunt or gather everything we eat, build shelters repeatedly, walk/run long distances, go for long periods without food, etc.

Our bodies *are doing what they've evolved to do*. It's our lives and especially our food that has changed so dramatically.

Ultra-Processed Foods, Drinks, Sugar, Addiction and the Brain

Ultra-processed foods/drinks and sugar are unique in their effects on the human brain. As we discussed in the previous section, our bodies are adapted to use carbohydrate for immediate energy or to store it as fat to be used later in times of food scarcity.

For reasons covered in the last section, ultra-processed foods and drinks and especially sugar *are inherently addictive* because they activate the reward centers in our brains incredibly quickly, and we need eat higher amounts of them in order to get the same effects in our brains.

Evolutionary forces drive us to seek out sweet foods and foods that rapidly become sugar in our bodies because these foods are a chance to store fat—something that meant survival during the millions of years of our evolution.

This is the reason *we're all* vulnerable to the effects of carbohydrate and most especially to ultra-processed foods/drinks and sugar. Humans do not develop addiction to protein or fat the way we do to carbohydrate, especially to ultra-processed carbohydrates like refined sugar, flours, and starches that do not exist in nature.

However, given that more than 60% of the American diet is now comprised of these "foods," addiction has become very widespread. Again, our bodies have not changed; the food has. We can't override evolution or the human hormonal system and how our bodies respond to these substances.

What we can do is remove them from our diets. Addiction to these foods has also been *normalized and encouraged* in multiple ways especially through advertising, the snack food industry, and government feeding programs such as school meals that include ultra-processed foods and sugar, etc.

Sadly (and frighteningly) our national Dietary Guidelines for Americans (DGA)[6], the government's national nutrition policy in the U.S., *tells us* we must include refined and processed grains in our diets (i.e. grains stripped of their natural matrix) in order to be healthy, which is complete nonsense from a scientific perspective.

According to these guidelines, which were updated for 2020-2025, everyone should be eating 6 servings of grains per day, 50% of which should be *refined.* We do not need to eat addictive, highly refined and processed junk that rapidly metabolizes into sugar in order to be healthy. The premise is ridiculous and dangerous.

We do not need to eat addictive, highly refined and processed junk in order to be healthy if we're eating natural foods with their entire *matrix intact*—i.e. fiber, water, 3 types of fat, protein, micronutrients, etc.

We also do not need to be eating huge amounts of grains, 6 servings per day, that all **become sugar** in the human body— especially given that carbohydrate itself is completely optional in the human diet.

School feeding programs, for example, can serve donuts, chips, cookies, etc. and count these health-destroying foods as *permissible and healthy* based on the Dietary Guidelines for Americans. It's completely crazy, and it fosters addiction to ultra-processed foods and sugar in particular.

---

[6] U.S. Department of Agriculture and U.S. Department of Health and Human Services. Dietary Guidelines for Americans, 2020-2025. 9th Edition. December 2020. https://www.dietaryguidelines.gov/

Remember, we're wired as a species to seek out sweet foods, so we can't give this garbage to children and expect them to resist powerful evolutionary forces such as attraction to sweetness or the ways in which high levels of glucose from these foods affects their vulnerable brains, which will not be full developed until they're in the late twenties, which is how long it takes for the human brain to mature fully.

Essentially, our national dietary guidelines in the United States, which are emulated all over the world, are promoting addiction to ultra-processed foods as well as sugar, including in children.

The DGA also tell us we should be eating lots of fruits and that juice is an option in a healthy diet. No it is not—not for anyone who has any metabolic health problem, which is now 88% of American adults.

Given what sugar and fructose *actually do* in the human body, especially with regard to the liver and brain, we should not be overwhelming our bodies all day with sugar (grains) sugar (fruits) refined grains (a lot of sugar), juice (sucrose and fructose) etc. and focusing our meals on carbohydrate (sugar) in general.

The DGA are a significant reason Americans are so addicted to ultra-processed foods and sugar in any and all forms because a diet high in carbohydrate makes us hungrier, drives cravings for foods that spike blood sugar, and drives cravings for sweetness in general.

Remember, sweetness is extremely rare in nature, which means as species we're wired to seek it out because it's so unusual in nature. We can't change this deeply ancient drive in us; we have to change availability of sweet and ultra-processed foods, especially our food environments—in our homes, schools, hospitals, nursing homes, stores, etc.

How addictive are ultra-processed foods and sugar? They're incredibly addictive. In his recent book, **Hooked: Food, Free Will, and How the Food Giants Exploit Our Addictions**, Pulitzer-prizing winning journalist Michael Moss shows us that the faster something hits our reward circuitry in the brain, the stronger its impact:

"The smoke from cigarettes takes 10 seconds to stir the brain, but a touch of sugar on the tongue will do so in a little more than a half second, or six hundred milliseconds, to be precise," Moss notes. "That's nearly 20 times faster than cigarettes." "Measured in milliseconds, and the power to addict, nothing is faster than processed food in rousing the brain." The faster a substance hits the brain, the more likely we are to act compulsively and impulsively.

In a recent article the *NYT* explains that like cigarettes and cocaine, the ingredients in ultra-processed foods and drinks also come from naturally occurring plants and foods (e.g. grains, sugar, starches). [7]

However, as we saw in the NOVA categories, these foods are then stripped of components that slow their absorption by the human body, such as fiber, water and protein. This is the reason these substances spike blood sugar and insulin levels so dramatically.

Ultra-processing means that these pleasurable ingredients are refined and processed into products that *are rapidly absorbed into the bloodstream*. This processing increases the capacity of these pleasurable ingredients to light up areas of our brains that regulate reward, emotion, and motivation.

---

[7] Anahad O'Connor. "Unhealthy Foods Aren't Just Bad For You, They May Also be Addictive." *The New York Times.* February 18, 2021: https://www.nytimes.com/2021/02/18/well/eat/food-addiction-fat.html

This means ingredients such as flours, starches, and sugars in their most concentrated and refined forms in processed foods are absorbed into the bloodstream very quickly and they are designed to affect multiple areas of our brains extremely quickly.

Ultra-processed food and drink manufacturers know this science; they know exactly how their products work. They know they're cultivating addiction and ruining our health. They use "calories" and the rhetoric of getting enough exercise to deflect their cultivation of addiction. ("Calories" don't cause addiction; the body has no receptors for calories.)

Like cigarettes and cocaine, their ingredients are derived from naturally occurring plants and foods that are stripped of the things that slow their absorption such as fiber, water, fat, and protein. Then their most pleasurable ingredients are refined and heavily processed into "foods" and drinks that are rapidly absorbed into the bloodstream, which enhances their ability to light up regions of the brain that regulate reward, emotion and motivation.

Salt, various thickeners and artificial flavors and other additives in ultra-processed processed foods and drinks strengthen their appeal and pull on us by enhancing texture and "mouth-feel," which is very similar to the ways in which cigarettes contain many additives designed to increase their addictiveness.

What's happening is that ultra-processed "foods" and drinks are being engineered to trigger the brain's "on switch" (mostly the neurotransmitter, dopamine) and inhibit its "off switch" (a region called the prefrontal cortex).[8] Ultra-processed foods often contain large amounts of fat, primarily in the form of toxic (and

---

[8] Daniel E. Lieberman. "The Science Behind Your Need for One More Potatoe Chip." *The New York Times.* March 12, 2021. https://www.nytimes.com/2021/03/12/books/review/hooked-michael-moss.html

cheap) "vegetable" oils, and refined carbohydrates, which is a combination that is *extremely rare* in the natural and real foods that humans evolved over millions of years eating: animal meat and animal fat, vegetables, beans and seeds, fruits.

Whole foods are high in either fat or carbohydrate, not both.

Thus, ultra-processed foods and drinks combine things— sweetness and saltiness, fat and carbs—that trick our hormones and hormonal signals (insulin and leptin in particular) while manipulating our taste buds and the reward centers in our brains.

Our bodies are deceived because ultra-processed foods and drinks exploit inherent evolutionary vulnerabilities we have as a species for both sweetness and fat, and the makers of these substances know this evolutionary biology all too well. Their profits depend on knowing it—and abusing it.

They also know that we need to keep increasing the "dose" of ultra-processed foods and sugar to get the same effects in the brain. Researches have found in brain imaging studies[9] that people who frequently consume ultra-processed foods and drinks ("junk food") can develop a tolerance to them over time, leading them to require larger and larger amounts to get the same enjoyment.

This is how addictive substances work. Food companies have deliberately engineered these ultra-processed foods and drinks to takeover the reward circuitry in our brains; doing so causes us to overeat and to experience chronic cycles of cravings that continue to worsen over time.

---

[9] Burger KS, Stice E. Frequent ice cream consumption is associated with reduced striatal response to receipt of an ice cream-based milkshake. Am J Clin Nutr. 2012 Apr;95(4):810-7. doi: 10.3945/ajcn.111.027003. Epub 2012 Feb 15. PMID: 22338036; PMCID: PMC3302359.

We don't choose these consequences—i.e. the ways in which these substances affect us for evolutionary reasons; this isn't a matter of personal choice but of biochemistry, neurochemistry, and hormonal responses. We don't control how the evolutionary adaptations of our species work. We don't control the anatomy of the human brain or how our hormonal system works, etc.

These foods are so profitable *because* they are addictive; the companies that make them know this, but do everything possible to shift the blame for their toxins to the individual.

This tactic is hardly new. It's the deflection and diversion at the core of the tobacco industry. The ultra-processed foods/drink industry and the tobacco industry are *not separate industries.* The tobacco industry started buying processed food and drink companies in the 1960's.

In their excellent 2019 article in the *BMJ*, "Tobacco industry involvement in children's sugary drinks,"[10] Nguyen et al. gives us a window into this relationship between tobacco companies and processed food/drink manufacturers. For example, Tobacco giant R.J. Reynolds led the transition to sweetened beverages in 1963 when it purchased Hawaiian Punch from Pacific Hawaiian Products Company, 1983, R.J. Reynolds introduced the nation's first juice box.

This juice box innovation was largely responsible for a 34 percent jump in sales, according to industry documents. Juices are high in sugar and fructose, and they are integral to getting kids to crave more and more sweetness and sugar.

Tobacco competitor Philip Morris had acquired Kool-Aid, via General Foods, in 1985. The company moved to marketing to children with its "Kool-Aid Man" mascot and launched

[10] *BMJ* 2019; 364 doi: https://doi.org/10.1136/bmj.l736 (Published 14 March 2019) BMJ 2019;364:l736

collaborations with branded toys such as Barbie and Hot Wheels. It also developed a children's Kool-Aid loyalty program described as "our version of the Marlboro Country Store," which was a cigarette incentives program. "The industry claims that these tobacco-inspired marketing strategies are not actually targeting children."

Ultra-processed foods companies also started buying diet companies in the late 1970s—i.e. to help us lose the weight caused by eating their toxic products. In a useful article in the *NYT*,[11] we learn that Heinz, the processed food giant, bought Weight Watchers in 1978; Unilever, which sells Klondike bars and Ben & Jerry's ice cream, bought SlimFast in 2000.

Nestle, which makes chocolate bars and Hot Pockets, purchased Jenny Craig in 2006. In 2010 the company that owns Cinnabon and Carvel ice cream purchased Atkins Nutritionals, which sells low-carb products. Philip Morris acquired Kraft and General Foods, making it the largest manufacturer of processed foods in the country with products like Kool-Aid, Jell-O, Chips Ahoy, and Oreo cookies.

Unfortunately, much of our nutrition science, including its educational institutions, is funded and deeply influenced by ultra-processed food and drink companies as well as drug companies. There is enormous resistance to changing our national dietary guidelines so they actually reflect the robust science on the nutritional needs of Americans.

Politics, influence, lobbying, and money, not science, are the forces behind our national nutrition policy that's telling us to eat dangerous ultra-refined and processed foods, far too much sugar, and far too much optional carbohydrate in general.

---

[11] Anahad O'Connor. "This is Your Brain on Junk Food." *The New York Times*. March 25, 2021: https://www.nytimes.com/2021/03/25/well/eat/hooked-junk-food.html

Ultra-processed foods and drinks are profoundly addictive. Despite our nonsensical, unscientific national dietary guidelines, these substances have little to no nutritional value even if they're "enriched" because we *can and should* be getting our micronutrients from whole foods, not cheap, synthesized vitamins and minerals, which may not be very bioavailable to humans, which are added back to these products after they've been stripped of their entire food matrix.

The DGA are also *nutritionally incomplete*, but that's a different story; suffice it to say, even if you follow the DGA *exactly*, you will still be eating a *nutritionally incomplete diet*. National dietary guidelines and nutrition policy about what's healthy to eat should not be nutritionally *in*complete, to say the least....

There is also no reason our dietary guidelines as a country should be telling us it's perfectly healthy to eat up to 10% of our diet in sugar—for *which the human body has exactly zero nutritional need.*

Given that there is *no nutritional need* for sugar, sugar should not be in these dietary guidelines at all because nutrition policies and dietary guidelines should be based on what people need to consume and avoid in order to be healthy.

Sugar is at *the top* of list of things to avoid given what it does to the human body and how toxic and addictive it is—and the 10% figure is total nonsense, not science.

That's supposed to be the entire point of the Dietary Guidelines for Americans that nearly all dieticians, nutritionists, MD's and everyone else in healthcare field are obligated to use when working with patients.

These are policies handed down to us; they're not merely idle ideas. Why does the DGA also say that 10% of our diet can be sugar—to please the ultra-processed food/drinks and sugar industries that fund so much of our nutrition science through research, grants, speaking engagements, perks and all the rest of it.

No wonder the ultra-processed food and drink companies are *doing everything possible* and pouring enormous amounts of money into lobbying in order to keep the status quo when it comes to maintaining our current national nutrition policy that tells Americans (and the world) it's not only safe—but it's healthy—to eat toxic, highly addictive substances—including ultra-processed foods and sugar.

These guidelines also determine what millions of Americans *can* eat—i.e. are able to eat—in schools, hospitals, nursing homes, the military, and in feeding programs for the most economically needy who are at *highest risk* of diet-related diseases and conditions.

Remember, "calories" are *pure deflection* designed to blame the individual for being affected by toxic substances in ways that are rooted in millions of years of evolutionary history and adaptations.

Processed food and beverage companies rely heavily on the nonsense about "calories"—as does the Dietary Guidelines for Americans to keep the profits from ultra-processed foods, drinks, and sugar rolling in.

"Personal choice" is intentionally deceptive rhetoric deployed to provide cover for theultra-processed food and drink giants and distance them from the devastating population-level consequences of their toxins on human health—i.e. the widespread metabolic diseases and conditions caused by their products. Finally, nutrition science itself tells us these substances are an essential part of being "healthy."

Many dieticians, nutritionists, and MD's may tell you that the Dietary Guidelines for Americans do not tell us to eat ultra-processed foods; *if one actually reads the DGA,* particularly the edict that one should consume *50% of one's 6 servings of grains per day as refined* (that's the word the DGA uses), eating very addictive, ultra-processed food is exactly what the DGA tells us to do because refined *means ultra-processed.*

Here's a graphic (below) of this instruction to eat half of your (far too many) servings of grains per day as ultra-processed grains in order to be healthy, which you can find on page 20 of the Dietary Guidelines for Americans 2020-2025.[12]

This is why kids in schools can eat ultra-processed foods—and the contracts for those foods and drinks in schools are massively lucrative; the U.S. government should not be acting, essentially, as a pusher creating and perpetuating addiction to toxic, addictive substances, including sugar, under the guise of healthy eating—all to ensure the *massive* profits of ultra-processed food/drinks and sugar companies.

(Expert advisors, who recommended reducing sugar and alcohol intake further, i.e. reducing two addictive toxins and poisons that have no nutritional value of any kind, were ignored when the 2020-2025 DGA were cobbled together from a toxic stew of funding, politics, and recalcitrance.)

---

[12] U.S. Department of Agriculture and U.S. Department of Health and Human Services. Dietary Guidelines for Americans, 2020-2025. 9th Edition. December 2020. https://www.dietaryguidelines.gov/

Table 1-1

Healthy U.S.-Style Dietary Pattern at the 2,000-Calorie Level, With Daily or Weekly Amounts From Food Groups, Subgroups, and Components

FOOD GROUP OR SUBGROUP	Daily Amount[b] of Food From Each Group (Vegetable and protein foods subgroup amounts are per week.)
Vegetables (cup eq/day)	2 ½
	Vegetable Subgroups in Weekly Amounts
Dark-Green Vegetables (cup eq/wk)	1 ½
Red and Orange Vegetables (cup eq/wk)	5 ½
Beans, Peas, Lentils (cup eq/wk)	1 ½
Starchy Vegetables (cup eq/wk)	5
Other Vegetables (cup eq/wk)	4
Fruits (cup eq/day)	2
Grains (ounce eq/day)	6
Whole Grains (ounce eq/day)	≥ 3
Refined Grains (ounce eq/day)	< 3

If you eat a diet of whole, unprocessed foods using the list of staples in **Section II** of this book—including animal products for important vitamins and fats that are only available in animal products—you do not need to eat any refined or ultra-processed grains for cheap, synthetic vitamins that your body may not absorb properly.

If you are vegan or vegetarian, you do need to supplement properly because these diets are nutritionally incomplete due to our evolutionary history as a species and how differently we absorb key vitamins from animal products vs. plant sources.

You can purchase *high-quality* supplements instead of relying on cheap, refined, ultra-processed foods for necessary vitamins such as the B complex vitamins, especially B12. Eating enough natural sources of fat is especially important so that you can absorb fat-soluble vitamins.

If you would like further resources for understanding processed food addiction as well as medical, historical, and critical perspectives of ultra-processed foods/drinks, see

Joan Ifland, Ph.D., M.B.A. *Processed Food Addiction*

Robert H. Lustig, M.D., M.S.L.: *Metabolical: The Lure and Lies of Processed Food, Nutrition, and Modern Medicine*

Michael Moss, *Hooked: Food, Free Will, and How the Food Giants Exploit Our Addictions*

Establishing Your Priorities

Prioritize taking the time you need to get rid of the **ultra-processed foods/drinks** and sugar in your home because these are the substances that cause chronic metabolic diseases and conditions including weight gain, Type 2 diabetes, NAFLD and drive cardiovascular disease and dementia.

They are the most addictive substances in our diets. They drive hunger. They cause cravings. They have next to no nutritional value. They are exceedingly expensive both directly and indirectly in terms of the health problems they cause.

When we limit or eliminate ultra-processed foods and drinks, we're going to automatically reduce our carbohydrate intake. Low sugar and low carbohydrate eating is a continuum, and eliminating ultra-processed foods and drinks is one point on this continuum. At the most strict end are the keto and carnivore diets.

One doesn't need to follow these diets necessarily in order to gain enormous health benefits; however, once we have a damaged carbohydrate metabolism from consuming ultra-processed foods/drinks over time, a specifically low-carbohydrate diet is what stabilizes blood sugar and insulin levels and affects the cellular pathways of insulin resistance, which no drug/medication can. As we've discussed, insulin resistance is what drives so many of our chronic health problems.

Begin by eliminating as many ultra-processed foods and drinks *and substituting them for whole, natural, and minimally processed foods and drinks*. Doing so is the single most important step in reversing cravings for ultra-processed foods and drinks. This takes some time, but the cravings become much easier to manage when we're eating a diet of whole (i.e. real) foods.

A key reason we have these cravings is because these substances cause *severe spikes in blood sugar and insulin levels*; when blood sugar starts to go down again, we seek foods that will spike it once more. When blood sugar drops but insulin stays high (insulin resistance / hyperinsulinemia, the cravings are especially difficult to manage.

Within a few weeks, you'll be very surprised by how much your tastes have changed eating a diet of whole and real foods; sweet foods, including fruits, become *unbearably* sweet, and ultra-processed foods taste unpalatable and unpleasant.

Our tastes change because we're *returning* to our normal sense of taste that's been distorted and abused by ultra-processed foods and their manufacturers. It takes time for our tastes to change, but they will. Whole, natural, real and unprocessed foods are *far more filling*, stabilize blood sugar and insulin secretion, improve blood pressure, and decrease appetite.

As you eat more of these whole and natural foods and eliminate ultra-processed foods and drinks, you'll find that *you're also far less hungry*, your cravings go way down, and it's much easier to choose healthy alternatives. You'll also find that stressors become easier to manage in relation to food choices.

The human body recognizes whole, unprocessed foods at the hormonal level because we evolved over millions of years eating these foods, so our brains get the hormonal signal, **leptin**, that we're full and to stop eating.

Keep in mind when insulin levels are high in the body, the brain doesn't "see" leptin, which means chronically high insulin levels prevent our brains from getting the hormonal message, leptin, which governs energy balance. We don't know that we're full.

Ultra-processed foods and drinks are fabricated to ensure these foods/drinks *evade our hormonal signals* so we'll keep eating them, especially when we're stressed. These foods are *designed to be addictive.*

This addiction process is *built into* these ultra-processed foods and drinks, and the manufacturers rely on the inherent addictiveness of these foods/drinks to make massive profits (while telling us it's all about "calories" in order to hide what they're doing). Addiction is *intentional and deliberate* when it comes to ultra-processed foods and drinks and their manufacturers.

Given the reality of how addictive ultra-processed foods and drinks are, it takes time to reduce and eliminate the amount of ultra-processed foods and drinks you consume.

It also takes time to learn to shop for and prepare unprocessed as well as minimally-processed foods such as meat, cheese, seafood, nuts and seeds, whole fruit (low-sugar) and whole vegetables (low-starch.)

You can go at your own pace; *each and every step you take makes a difference over time.* This is about permanent change, not a crash diet.

It's about eating for health for the rest of your life, and if it takes time to remove these dangerous substances from your life, take the time you need. Know that the cravings will decrease substantially for ultra-processed foods and sugar as you focus your diet on whole and real foods.

Consider Keeping a Food Journal

Ultra-processed foods and drinks now constitute the **majority of the American diet—60%**, which is why, as a population, we're so sick with chronic metabolic diseases and conditions such as prediabetes and Type 2 diabetes, obesity, hypertension, and cholesterol problems.

Ultra-processed foods and drinks, especially sugar and high levels of fructose in processed foods and drinks, are the primary cause of these chronic metabolic health problems.

By causing insulin resistance over time, these foods and drinks drive a wide range of diseases and conditions, some of which we've discussed in previous sections, including, nonalcoholic fatty liver disease (NAFLD), weight gain, prediabetes and Type 2 diabetes, hypertension, cholesterol problems and the cluster of diet-driven problems known as Metabolic Syndrome.

Eating too many "calories," or meat and fat are not the problem. It's all the highly refined grains, starches, and sugars in ultra-processed foods and drinks that are driving the epidemic of poor metabolic health, including weight problems that are now endemic in the American population.

They are highly addictive because they are manufactured to be addictive so we'll keep eating and drinking them.

It's the sugar, bad fats ("vegetable" oils), and highly refined carbohydrates in these ultra-processed foods that affect our brains in highly addictive ways, particularly the sugar.

It can be very helpful to track your cravings and consumption of ultra-processed foods and sugar in all forms, including fruit and juices. Doing so on a daily basis will help you better understand your carbohydrate cravings, which is what most ultra-processed foods are, so you can make better choices each day.

Given that ultra-processed foods/drinks and sugar are so addictive, tracking your cravings in response to stressors in your life is particularly important.

Once you can better identify how specific stressors or triggers prompt cravings for ultra-processed foods/drinks/sugar, the better able you will be to make healthy choices. Keep in mind that limiting/eliminating ultra-processed foods/drinks and sugar isn't about perfection; it's a process.

Remember, all ultra-processed foods/drinks become sugar (glucose) *very* quickly in the body, even if they don't contain much "added" sugar. These foods have little to no fiber, so our bodies convert them to sugar (glucose) rapidly.

This produces a sugar rush—spike in blood sugar—with the corresponding spike in insulin—even if there isn't much "added" sugar in the foods.

Sugar in ultra-processed foods and drinks excite brain cells—i.e. we get a sugar rush—before *sugar kills brain cells*. Sugar is very toxic to the brain as well as to the heart and the immune system.

However, all ultra-processed foods/drinks cause a sugar rush as well; salty or savory ultra-refined carbohydrates such as chips, crackers, most bread, etc. and other savory ultra-processed foods and snacks that are lower in added sugar than candy or ice cream *still become sugar* in the human body. To the body, *all these things are sugar and more sugar*—causing spikes in insulin response.

When insulin stays high but blood sugar crashes after eating these foods, we become "hangry" and experience worsening food cravings for more ultra-processed foods/drinks that will spike blood sugar again quickly. It's a vicious cycle that gets

---

exponentially worse over time affecting our weight, blood sugar, blood pressure, cholesterol, inflammation levels, heart, and brain health.

One of the other very toxic ingredients in most ultra-processed "foods" is "vegetable" oils, which *don't come from vegetables.* They are highly toxic; essentially, they're light machine oils, which was their original use before they were put into the food supply as a way to make profits from the waste products of other industries.

The human body can't metabolize these light machine oils properly, and they are especially dangerous for the cardiovascular system. Their toxic byproducts get buried in the endothelial lining of the vascular system damaging our arteries and hearts.

These oils include soybean, canola, safflower, corn, grape seed, rapeseed, cottonseed, etc. (Olive oil does not fall into this category, nor does coconut oil, neither of which come from beans or seeds.)"Vegetable" oils (a.k.a. light machine oils) are widely used in ultra-processed foods because they're very cheap.

So, when you're limiting or eliminating ultra-processed foods, you're also limiting or eliminating many sources of these toxic "vegetable" oils that damage our hearts and brains in particular. Go back to using butter, cheese, and if you eat it, meat.

Do not use spreads that contain a mixture of olive oil/butter and vegetable oils such as soybean or canola; they're marketed to give us the idea we're getting the taste of butter while getting the "benefits" of "vegetable" oils—i.e. fewer calories, etc. Use olive oil and coconut oil if you're vegetarian or vegan.

For salad dressings, which are a major source of these toxic oils, make your own dressings at home with a good olive oil and vinegar of your choice, herbs, lemon, etc. It only takes a minute to whip up a delicious dressing.

Making your own dressings at home is also considerably cheaper than buying toxic "vegetable" oil dressings in stores. You can keep your dressing in the fridge, and just put it on the counter for the olive oil to soften before use. You can also put in microwave for a few seconds—just enough to melt the olive oil but not heat the dressing.

Remember, the human species evolved eating a diet of animal products—meat, seafood, and the natural sources of fat in these foods, which contain all 3 types of fat together—so our bodies metabolize and respond extremely well to these foods in their natural and minimally processed forms.

Our genes, cells, hormones, etc. "understand" these foods because we spent millions of years during our evolutionary history consuming them. For millions of years during which 99% of our genes were established, we didn't eat light machine oils ("vegetable" oils)—i.e. before the invention of the machinery these oils were created to lubricate. These oils work very well in machinery, but their molecular structure is a serious problem for the human body.

If you decide to keep a journal, there are many types and styles available in a variety of formats to suit your purposes. I created a journal specifically for people who want to limit or eliminate ultra-processed foods and sugar that you might find helpful: *The Processed Food & Sugar Elimination Journal*. You can easily create your own journal using prompts that work best to help you track and better understand your relationship to ultra-processed foods and sugar.

Summary of Health Implications of Sugar and Ultra-Processed Foods and Drinks

1.) Carbohydrate, most especially ultra-processed foods and sugar, spikes blood sugar and insulin levels the most. Ultimately, excess glucose gets stored as fat. High levels of insulin in the body cause insulin resistance and hyperinsulinemia over time leading to prediabetes/Type 2 diabetes and weight gain along with blood pressure and cholesterol problems.

As these conditions worsen, we develop cardiovascular disease, NAFLD, and dementia. These are diet- driven diseases and conditions in the vast majority of cases.

2.) *Dietary fat does not make us fat.* We *need* natural sources of fat for critical functions throughout the body. The dangerous fats are "vegetable" oils that we're told to eat by most dietary authorities. These are made from seeds and beans, and their original use was as machine oils. They were put into the human food supply in order to make profits from the waste products of other industries.

The crops from which these come, especially soy and corn, are heavily subsidized in the U.S., and the governmental agency co-responsible for our national dietary guidelines and nutrition policy, the USDA, is also responsible for promoting these crops. It's a profound conflict of interest that's harming our health.

3.) Ultra-processed and refined carbs as well as natural sources of sugar such as fruit, honey, etc. are *all highly addictive* and *increase hunger.*

As a species we're driven to seek our very rare sweet foods because they were so rare in nature, and they gave our bodies the rare opportunity to spike blood glucose and store that extra glucose as energy for later—as fat.

We're driven to do the same with uncommon sources of carbohydrate in nature (e.g. seasonal plants and berries) because they're an opportunity to store fat via temporary insulin resistance, which our evolution as a species prioritizes.

Ultra-processed foods/drinks deliberately exploit and target these vulnerabilities in our evolutionary history through isolated ingredients such as refined grains, flours, starches and sugar, ingredients stripped of all their natural food matrices.

This means these "foods" and drinks spike blood sugar quickly, affect the brain rapidly, trick our hormone leptin so we don't know we're full when we eat these substances, and cause permanent insulin resistance.

These spikes in blood sugar and stimulation of the reward centers in our brains often mean we can turn to ultra-processed foods/drinks and sugar to manage emotions, deal with stress, and to celebrate achievements/socialize. Our bodies have not changed in terms of our evolutionary history; what changed are our food environments and social norms.

This means we're consuming enormous quantities of these foods / drinks in our daily lives and for a wide range of reasons that have been encouraged and promoted, including by our national dietary guidelines that tell us we should eat ultra-processed and refined grains—3 servings per day for reasons that are deeply _un_scientific.

4.) Reducing ultra-processed foods/drinks and sugar is challenging given the central role they play in all areas of our lives and because these substances are designed to affect our biochemistry, hormones, and neurochemistry in ways that lie in evolutionary history, not personal willpower.

It's also difficult to reduce them because of convenience and because the medical and nutrition science establishments still tell us we need to consume high amounts of carbohydrate when this is *factually untrue.*

5.) *Humans do not need to consume any carbohydrate* provided we eat enough protein and fat. The liver makes all the glucose our brains need via *gluconeogenesis.*

6.) All carbohydrate is addictive to some degree, but ultra-processed foods/drinks and sugar are manufactured to be highly addictive to humans. This is deliberate because it's very profitable to keep people addicted to these substances.

7.) Ultra-processed foods and drinks have little to no nutritional value, and the nutritional requirement for sugar in the human diet is zero—none.

8.) Focus on eliminating *ultra-processed* foods and drinks by eating more nutrient-dense protein, natural sources of fat such as meat, fish, full-fat dairy and cheese, as well as non-starchy vegetables and limited low-sugar fruits.

9.) You must replace ultra-processed foods and drinks and sugar with natural and whole foods that will make you full and satisfied because these foods align with our hormonal and digestive systems that evolved over millions of years as we ate these whole and natural foods.

10.) Natural fat such as olive oil, avocados, nuts and seeds, dairy, butter, meats, fish, etc. make us far more satisfied, so we end up eating less while we are getting more of what we need nutritionally.

These are the kinds of fats the human body metabolizes properly, *not corn, soybean, canola or other similar "vegetable" or "plant-based" oils* that are the *byproducts* of other industries and fabricated through intensive industrial and chemical processes.

Natural fat like butter takes about 18 hours for the body to process; dangerous, chemical, unstable "vegetable" oils (excluding olive and coconut oils, which are fine) take about 60days to process, and still cause significant harm in the brain, heart, and vascular system.

11.) It's close to *impossible to overeat* protein and fat because our bodies always tell us when we're full when we eat protein and fat. On the other hand, ultra-processed foods/drinks and sugar, especially sugar in any form including sugary fruits, make us *increase hunger.*

Carbs with high sugar/starch such as potatoes, rice, wheat, and corn etc. *trigger hunger.* Eating a lot of fruit makes us hungrier because of the sugar in it. Sucrose (table sugar) and all the other forms of sugar in ultra-processed foods and drinks make us *the most* hungry.

Sugar and ultra-processed foods = hunger
Natural sources of fat, protein, and fiber = feeling satisfied

12.) *It takes time* to limit or eliminate ultra-processed foods/drinks and sugar and to work through the very real effects of ultra-processed food and sugar addiction and withdrawal if these are applicable to you. The progress you make *over time* is what matters.

Replacing each ultra-processed food or drink with a natural, whole food is the goal.

You can buy or create a journal as a tool to help you understand your cravings for ultra-processed foods/drinks and sugar, most especially the triggers and stressors that can cause us to reach for these foods.

Replacing ultra-processed foods/drinks and sugar with whole and natural foods is a process, one that will utterly transform your health and your relationship to food. Limiting/eliminating these substances (remember, they're *not* food) can be challenging, and there will be setbacks.

Take the time you need to move toward a diet of whole and natural foods at the pace you can. Know that *every* step you take matters, and every step makes a difference to your health and wellness.

Section II:

Shopping, Organizing, Preparing: Cooking All Your Meals For A Week in 2 Hours

Food Staples, Grocery Lists, and Ingredients

The first step is to focus on throwing out all the ultra-processed and items with sugar that you have in the house. If they're in the house, it becomes far more difficult to resist them.

This step is key. If it comes in a box, package, jar, or bottle, use the *NOVA classification system*[13] to determine if it's a natural food, a processed food, or an ultra-processed one. In particular, if you're trying to manage cravings for ultra-processed foods and/or sugar, it's crucial not to have any of these foods or drinks in the house.

The next step is to shop for appropriate foods, which we'll discuss below. The third step is to begin a weekly cooking routine. Below is a list of staples that will form the foundation of a natural/whole foods diet.

Remember that fat is essential to all humans, and you should be sure to include adequate sources of natural fats such as butter, cheese, olive oil, coconut oil, fatty cuts of meat, chicken with the skin on, and fish.

---

[13] Monteiro CA, Cannon G, Moubarac JC, Levy RB, Louzada MLC, Jaime PC. The UN Decade of Nutrition, the NOVA food classification and the trouble with ultra-processing. *Public Health Nutr.* 2018 Jan;21(1):5-17. doi: 10.1017/S1368980017000234. Epub 2017 Mar 21. PMID: 28322183.

Food Staples are the items you always have and from which you can make all your meals. This list isn't very long because eating real, whole, and natural foods that are nutritionally complex and satisfying to eat means you have *ingredients* in the house, not prepared foods.

Having a house full of ingredients means you are now a connoisseur of food, a culinary adventurer!

Getting rid of all the ultra-processed and prepared foods and sugar means saving a lot of money *and* you have a great opportunity to try new things and new cuisines.

Don't be intimidated! Great chefs experiment; it's what makes them great chefs.

You don't need a lot of ingredients to make many kinds of fantastic meals with genuine variety, and these meals don't need to take a lot of time to prepare.

Spending a couple of hours a week prepping food is absolutely crucial. *Food prep* is the key to everything, which we'll discuss. Let's discuss the basic staples that form the foundation of a natural, whole food diet.

Basic Staples

Lentil or bean low-sodium soups in boxes or cans without BPA lining and no pastas, added sugar, chemicals, etc. The organic brands are far more likely not to include these things. You can extend these with rinsed canned beans and chopped veggies, broth, and herbs for soup that's fast and easy to make. Add the meat and veggies you like, just use several kinds of veggies so you have a range of tastes, textures, and nutrients.

If you like you can add some chicken or veggie broth, garlic, a good herb mixture, a little Parmesan cheese and olive oil, and you're all set. Using a can of lentil or bean soup gives you the foundation for making complex, rich stews that are satisfying and economical—not to mention very nutritious.

Fruit that's lower on the glycemic index such as berries, tomatoes, avocados, lemons and limes. Lemons can be used in a variety of ways in cooking to bring brightness to a dish and provide valuable vitamin C without the sugar.

Dairy such as creamer, butter, cheese, etc. Be very careful of yogurt. Even many "natural" yogurts have added sugar, fruit juice, etc., and there's a high level of natural sugar in milk/yogurt.

Don't eat low fat yogurt—it has a high level of natural sugar without the fat to slow the absorption of that sugar. Include some full fat dairy such as cheese and heavy cream in your coffee. Remember, natural sources of fat are *essential* in the human diet, and they are uniquely satisfying—which helps decrease cravings for ultra-processed foods and sugar.

If you are dairy intolerant, you can substitute **unsweetened** nut milks and products. Be extremely careful of dairy alternatives that use soy or soybean oil because of the way vegetable oils adversely affect the human cardiovascular system and brain. These are not healthy foods.

If you are dairy intolerant, focus on getting your healthy fats from fish, meat, olive oil, coconut oil, avocados, nuts and seeds, and nut butters that are not hydrogenated—i.e. the oil will be floating at the top because this is natural when products are not hydrogenated. Make sure your nut or seed butters do not have sweeteners.

Meat (e.g. chicken, red meat, turkey, organ meats)

Canned tomatoes for making many kinds of dishes.

Broth, low sodium if you prefer, for soups and to use as flavoring in dishes. (If you can, freeze the bones from your meats and make your own broth. If you have a slow cooker, this is easy to do, and you get all the minerals from the bones.)

Mushrooms, which are *powerful* immune boosters—even the plain white button mushrooms!

Beans/legumes—dried or canned without BPA lining to make soups, chili, use in sauces for extra fiber, to make cold bean salads with chopped veggies, etc.

Eggs

Nuts and Seeds, Nut Butters Without hydrogenated oils

Whole Grains such as quinoa that you make at home. Bob's Red Mill has many options.

Greens—use the boxed or bagged kind, and the Olivia's brand is organic and hasn't had the e-coli problem that other brands of greens have had. Supermarkets use chemicals in the sprayers over the produce section. Boxes/bags protect the greens.

Hummus

Veggies, organic whenever possible, and buy seasonally for better deals. Never eat conventional celery or red peppers or broccoli or kale—they are some of the worst and most toxic crops sprayed heavily with pesticides—eat only organic with these.

Focus on a range of colors and veggies that grow above ground because they have far less starch (sugar) so they are less likely to trigger cravings for sweetness or spike your blood sugar/insulin levels. You should have enough veggies to eat at lunch and dinner.

Don't forget about **frozen veggies**, which have good nutritional profiles. Peas, onions, organic broccoli, etc. are all great frozen choices because you can just add them to soups without chopping. Having a variety in the freezer always means you have things to add to soups or to other dishes. Use peas and onions in moderation as they have more starch.

Always have garlic and herbs on hand to add to soups and a variety of dishes. If garlic is too pungent, you can roast whole cloves along with your veggies/meat/ fish, and that way you can spread it on the final dish. Roasted garlic has a more mellow taste.

Using crushed garlic in soups adds to the robustness, and if you don't use a lot, it won't take over the flavor profile. You can roast a whole, red onion as a vegetable and makes a wonderful side for meat or beans.

Quinoa, Chia Seeds, and Ground flax for fiber and omega 3 fatty acids. Quinoa is a complete protein; it is high in carbohydrate, so think of it as a condiment rather than a main dish. Be sure to get ground flax seeds as humans can't digest whole flax seeds, so we don't get the benefits of the omega-3 fatty acids. Keep ground flax in the fridge in a dark bag or container.

This vegan source of omega-3 fatty acids is less bioavailable to the human body than animal products, so one should also supplement appropriately if one doesn't eat animal products.

Wild salmon whenever possible or other kinds of fatty fish such as sardines. Used canned wild salmon when fresh is out of season. When wild salmon is available in season and on sale, get extra to freeze. You can mix previously frozen wild salmon with an egg and herbs/seasoning of your choice to make wild salmon cakes that are great hot or cold.

I advise against farm-raised salmon, which does not have the same nutritional profile as wild salmon in terms of omega-3 fatty acids. Better to get wild on sale and freeze it to make salmon cakes later or used canned wild salmon.

Sardines make a fast, affordable snack or light meal that won't spike your blood sugar/insulin levels, so they don't cause food cravings. The fatty acids in them are important for our health and leave us feeling satisfied.

They provide lots of bioavailable calcium if you eat the bones. They're very economical and stay shelf stable for years. The wild sardines are best. They're also low on the food chain, so they're not building up mercury and other toxins in their flesh the way larger fish can such as tuna.

Herbs, dried or fresh. Some herbs such as oregano have far more antioxidants when dry. Think in terms of creating several herb mixes that you can put together in separate containers for quick use in creating a complex flavor profile to any dish, e.g. basil, oregano, thyme, rosemary and bay for dishes such as meatballs with chopped tomatoes, olive oil, and red onion.

A range of spice mixes and marinades, etc. that you like, which are low in sugar and salt. The **Teeny Tiny Spice Company** has an excellent line of organic spice mixes that you can just add quickly to meat, fish, or veggies to make a dish with a complex flavor profile without all the work.

They have choices of spice mixes from all over the world; these flavors add depth and interest to foods without the sugar, "vegetable" oils, salt and chemicals in marinades.

When cooking meats/fish these spices and seasonings will infuse the cooking liquid. If you're vegetarian or vegan, toss veggies with some water and fat (olive or coconut oil) into which you mix the spice blend of choice before cooking.

You can add a tablespoon or two of your favorite spice mix to unsweetened Greek yogurt to marinate chicken, fish, and meat, which adds calcium and fat—don't use low fat yogurt! Be sure to get yogurt that does not have any added sugar or sweeteners.

This homemade marinade should cling to the chicken or fish or meat so it's coated when it goes in the oven at 325 degrees.

This yogurt marinade ensures the chicken, or fish, or meat stays moist so you can cook a substantial amount ahead of time and just reheat quickly for subsequent meals, or slice for salads, etc.

Single-source olive oil and vinegars

Use the money you were spending on processed/prepared foods to get a single-source, extra-virgin organic olive oil. It will be more expensive, but it's a good fat that is stable at the molecular level when heated. If you eat animal products, get a good grass-fed butter as well for cooking and finishing dishes.

Try different vinegars. As a fermented food, vinegar has real health benefits, particularly for gut health. There are good quality options that are worth the money, and you will be saving money when you don't purchase processed/prepared foods.

Weekly Food Prep and Cooking

It's important to making cooking as easy and convenient as possible. The fast food and snack industries have made it *seem* as though cooking is far too time consuming when that just isn't true. You **don't** have to spend endless hours in the kitchen to make fantastic meals that are better than anything you can get in most restaurants—and for a fraction of the cost.

The key to having great meals all week that **take only minutes to assemble** throughout the week is to spend **a couple of hours each week doing all the prep, cooking, and clean up for the week**.

What takes so much time is prepping, cooking, and cleaning up after each meal—i.e. doing all these things scratch. Prepping, cooking, and cleaning up for 21 meals (breakfast, lunch, and dinner) during the week is incredibly time consuming because we're reinventing the wheel each time.

When you spend a couple of hours doing batch prep, cooking, and clean up for the entire week, you save an *enormous* amount of time—and you always have healthy foods to eat for breakfast, lunch, dinner, and healthy snacks. As you perfect this routine, your cutting/prep, organization, and cooking skills will improve significantly.

At first you might spend 3 hours per week preparing 21 meals per person for the week, 3 per day, until your skills and the routine of batch prep and cooking become second nature. Soon you'll get the routine down, and you can definitely do everything in two hours.

You can cut that time down further by having someone prep the veggies in advance. This weekly, organized food prep and cooking is an excellent way to teach children and teenagers many things.

These include how to take care of themselves, feed themselves, and develop good cooking skills. Most importantly when kids and teenagers and young adults are integral to food prep and cooking on a weekly basis, it teaches them how to avoid dangerous ultra-processed foods, drinks, and sugar that are marketed *intensively* to them.

Having the kids involved in prep and cooking saves time, but far more importantly, it saves their health and empowers them in profound ways.

Remember, **batch cooking once a week for two hours** gives you a week's worth of meals and drastically cuts down on shopping, prep, cooking, and clean up during the week. Breakfast and lunch become easy and inexpensive—and full of great food.

Because you're also **shopping for a week of meals**, you're also saving time by not having to go to the grocery store nearly as often.

Shopping for a week's worth of meals also ensures that you are focused on what you want your meals to be during the week, so you will be and will be less likely to buy impulse purchases or prepared meals that are usually highly processed.

When you come home hungry and tired from work, you don't have to deal with spending 30-60 minutes cooking and then another 30 minutes doing dishes and clean up.

If dinner is a matter of choosing from a wide range of great food that's ready to eat, you will be far less likely to eat processed, frozen dinners, or takeout for the convenience, because you already have convenient, delicious meals waiting for you—in your own fridge.

Dinner is just a matter of getting a plate and choosing the meat, veggies, and grain you want and heating! This is faster than takeout, delivery, or even a frozen dinner.

The sauces that you spent a couple of minutes reducing on the stovetop ensure that your dinners taste wonderful, and because you cooked with some water and didn't over cook your meat and veggies, your food will easily tolerate reheating in the microwave.

You'll have so many choices for protein and vegetables throughout the week that you can have a different breakfast, lunch, and dinner virtually every day. You'll be eating a delicious dinner in 5 minutes—delivery takes longer than that.

You can easily make a salad to go with your dinners by using boxed organic greens and a quick dressing you make with olive oil and vinegar.

You can add a side of hummus or bean salad made with 3 cans of rinsed beans and a good olive oil/vinegar dressing. Best of all, doing the dishes is a snap because you have *assembled* dinner, not made it from scratch each night.

In the next few pages you'll find directions for preparing all your meals for the week in advance.

> Before you get started, make sure you have an <u>empty dishwasher</u> so you can just load it as you go along during your *two hours of food prep per week*.
>
> Store your meats and fish in the fridge using the pans/dishes in which you cook them.

> <u>STEP ONE</u>: Prep and Cook your vegetables for the entire week. This should take about one hour to prep and cook all the veggies at one time depending on the size of your family. Choose a variety of vegetables you like, and take advantage of seasonal sales.

1.) **Cook one or two trays/big cooking dishes of cut veggies for the entire week depending on the size of your family.** This way you'll always have plenty of variety, sufficient micronutrients and fiber, and sufficient complex carbs for energy that don't spike blood sugar in the way ultra-processed foods and sugar do.

What takes so much time is all the prep—i.e. cutting vegetables each day and cooking them.

When you do all your chopping and cooking at once, you *save yourself a lot of energy and time during the week*. The key is not to overcook your veggies and to add a little water to keep them moist while cooking.

Leaving them slightly undercooked is best because you can soften them quickly in the microwave, heat as part of soup, or enjoy al dente as part of a salad or side dish.

2.) Chop roughly and toss your veggies with olive oil or butter and herbs, and cook in oven on **325 degrees** (not too hot), *with some water so they don't dry out.* Cook until just tender. You must add a good fat such as butter or olive oil because many vitamins are fat soluble, meaning we must eat fat in order to absorb them.

Cook dense veggies such as cauliflower, carrots, Brussels sprouts, broccoli, sweet potato, onions, etc. together on one tray and more fragile veggies such as peppers, mushrooms, tomatoes, asparagus, summer squash, etc. on another tray, as these two trays will be different cooking times.

These more fragile vegetables that have more water in them such as pepper, mushrooms, etc. *will take about 2/3 the cooking time* as the more dense, fibrous vegetables.

3.) You can also use a portion of your cut and prepped veggies in a stir-fry if you like—with spices and seasonings you like such as fresh ginger, garlic, chilies, and soy sauce—that you cook on the stove and garnish with cilantro or sesame seeds.

You should use a good olive oil or butter in which to cook you stir-fry.

You will be avoiding all the sugar and "vegetable" oils in restaurants, which are often reheated multiple times making them extremely toxic.

If you want, you can toss in some diced meat or fish in the last few minutes of cooking, and you'll have an amazing set of meals.

Uses for your veggies throughout the week:

1.) Mix with dressing (olive oil and vinegar—not soybean oil!!) for a cold dish.

2.) Add to a can of lentil or bean soup and garnish with olive oil for a robust one-dish meal

3.) Mix with some of your boxed organic greens for a complex salad that takes only a minute to prepare

4.) Serve with your protein, fish, chicken, or meat, along with a medley of vegetables for dinner along with a side of grains such as quinoa, or bean salad.

Prep one or two veggie tray bakes of veggies each week depending on the size of your family. When they're cooked and ready in the fridge, then it's just a matter of adding them to the meats, grains, or soups for an instant main dish.

You can cook one tray early in the week and cook the other tray of already-prepped vegetables later in the week if you like. What saves enormous time is *doing all your chopping and prep of your veggies at one time.* This also gives you an enormous variety of veggies to enjoy with each meal.

If you're vegetarian or vegan, you have the foundation of your meals ready to go with your pre-prepared/cooked veggies and genuine whole grain such as quinoa that you've cooked and stored in the fridge.

> **Step TWO:** *While your vegetables for the week are cooking for 30-45 minutes*, <u>make all your breakfasts</u> for the week.
>
> **Use individual containers that you have ready you have them all together in the fridge so you can just choose what you want and reheat in microwave.**

You should **focus on protein and fat** for breakfast to keep you full and limit blood sugar spikes, which cause hunger and drive cravings.

Options for breakfasts include:

1.) Cooking **a large batch of scrambled eggs or a large omelet**, enough for several servings depending on the size of your family—and to which you can add cooked veggies and meats later if you like when reheating. **Be sure to add** some water or cream to the beaten eggs before cooking, as these will keep them moist in the fridge and during reheating in microwave.

   Add melted cheese and herbs if you like. Cook in butter or olive oil. This is a robust and filling breakfast that won't leave you looking for a snack in the middle of the morning.

2.) **Prepare containers in advance with a serving size of whole, unsweetened yogurt** to which you add nuts, seeds, berries, etc. for a quick morning parfait that's economical and filling. I would recommend whole fat yogurt for three reasons: we need good fat, which is essential in the human diet; *low-fat yogurt is always sweetened* with honey, fruits, sugar, agave or other alternative sweeteners to compensate for the lack of fat; fat keeps us full and satisfied.

3.) **Prepare a batch of oatmeal** from scratch that's enough for several servings contingent upon the size of your family. **Use whole oats**, not instant oatmeal that is full of sugar and chemicals. You want the fiber in whole oats. As it cooks you can add nuts and seeds, butter, cream, berries, or flavors such as cinnamon.

Step THREE: Prepare and Cook Your Proteins for the Week

As you did in Step One and Step Two, you're going to prepare and cook all your proteins or main dishes at once: e.g. meats, chicken, and fish. If you are a vegetarian or vegan, this would be grains, beans, legumes, and other proteins such as tofu.

Put the dishes, silverware, cutting boards, etc. you use in the dishwasher *as you go along*, but store your meats/fish/proteins in the fridge in the oven dishes/containers in which you cooked them.

Prep all your meat, chicken, and fish for the week and cook at the same time in the oven at **325 degrees.** The principle is the same: batch cooking saves enormous amounts of time and you're not doing all the dishes from cooking separate meals each night.

Dinner becomes a matter of choosing from all the foods that are ready to go—i.e. a matter of getting a plate and choosing from a wide range of delicious, filling foods that are there waiting in your fridge—and quickly heating the plate in the microwave.

Options include:

1.) You can roast a whole chicken that you cut in half to speed up cooking; use butter or olive oil to seal in juices, rub with a spice mix you want, etc. or cook plain to use in several meals in different ways

2.) You can quickly make a batch of meatballs with garlic and herbs and bake in a dish with canned tomatoes and olive oil

3.) You can make a delicious meatloaf with one egg, herbs/seasonings of choice, garlic, some diced tomatoes from a can

4.) You can cook lamb chops or make lamb meatballs with seasonings

5.) You can cook cuts of beef or lamb on the stovetop, but cook just until done so they will withstand reheating.

6.) You can cook a pot roast in the oven or a large turkey breast, etc.

7.) Bake enough fish of choice for the week in the oven with lemon, garlic, white wine and herbs. **Put the fish closest to the oven door,** as it will be ready to take out first. Depending on the thickness of the cut and the type of fish, check at 20 minutes. Again, cook until just done.

In terms of meats such as **beef, pork, lamb** etc., bigger cuts save prep time and keep the meat moist during the week.
If you have an Instant Pot you can easily use that for one meat dish such as meatballs or a whole chicken while you're cooking the other meats/protein in the oven or making a bean soup/stew on the stovetop.

Just remember not to overcook your meat/fish because you want the meat to withstand reheating in the microwave as you assemble dinner plates throughout the week.

Once you take your meat, chicken, and fish out of the oven, **quickly reduce the liquids** in them in separate pans on the stove with spice mixes of your choice or red/white wine, butter and fresh herbs for robust sauces to pour over the finished meat/fish.

These reduced sauces take just a few minutes—you're just evaporating the water in the liquid and intensifying the flavors—and these sauces seal in all the flavors and moisture of your meats and fish. You can do these all at the same time in different pans and put them directly into the dishwasher.

While your proteins are cooking, make a grain you'd like to have on hand for the week such as quinoa. Make enough for the number of servings you'd like to have that week for dinner or lunches. If you have an Instant pot, quinoa cooks in **one minute**. You can use chicken, beef, or vegetable stock for better flavor. This is a matter of letting it cook for the designated time and stirring occasionally. When cool, you can just put the pot in which you cooked your grain in the fridge to add to dinners during the week.

Summary: Preparing and cooking food is **all about organization and using your two hours** in the kitchen per week effectively. You'll be doing all the work up front, and loading your dishwasher as you go along.

This means you're not reinventing the wheel—prepping, cooking, and cleaning up—for each of 21 meals (breakfasts, lunches, and dinners) each and every day. This is how you save so much time and make it much harder to give in to cravings for ultra-processed "convenient" foods.

When your breakfasts and lunches are all ready to grab-and-go, or heat and eat, you are far less likely to eat out or choose ultra-processed convenience foods because of hunger or temptation. *You've created all the convenience* inside your fridge!

Eat protein and fat for breakfast because it will keep you much more full and satisfied longer than ultra-processed (and expensive) breakfast cereals or breakfast bars, which increase hunger by spiking blood sugar. When our blood sugar drops after eating these, we become hungrier.

Protein and fat burn slowly like big logs on a fire giving us a steady, even source of energy; glucose/sugar from carbohydrate burns fast and intensely like paper, but the energy expires quickly leaving us hungry again—and more likely to eat another ultra-processed food that will spike blood sugar again. The energy we get from protein and fat start to wears off far more slowly and gradually.

This makes resisting processed foods/drinks and sugar *much* easier if we're not fighting severe swings in blood sugar—highs and drops—from the quick intense rushes of sugar from ultra-processed foods and drinks.

Organizing and Storing Your Prepared Meals

I would recommend that you dedicate one shelf in your fridge for **your prepared breakfasts and lunches** and one shelf for **your cooked proteins, grain(s), and your cooked vegetables**. That way you can find things quickly by meal.

Once you get this food prep and cooking routine down, you might cook slightly larger portions of meat, chicken, fish, veggies, beans/legumes and grains. As you did with your breakfasts and lunches, set aside a few containers to make **meals to put in your freezer**. It's very helpful to have 5-6 frozen, homemade meals in the freezer.

For example, if you can't go shopping for the week as you normally do, you have a few days of meals ready to eat, which makes it far less likely you'll order takeout or be tempted to eat processed/ultra-processed foods. If you're sick and can't do your weekly shopping/cooking, you have meals ready to go.

Finally if bad weather/storm storm is expected, everyone rushes to the grocery store. You can avoid this because you have meals all prepared in your fridge, or if you're almost done with your prepared meals in your fridge, you can weather the storm with your frozen meals and canned soups, nuts/seeds, and canned fish and meats that you should always have in your pantry.

Meatballs cooked in diced tomatoes and hers/garlic with olive oil freeze beautifully. For chicken, you can put it shredded cooked chicken into a container with veggies, grains, beans, etc. and some broth, and you'll have delicious chicken stew.

You can do the same with fish or lamb, etc. Bean soups/stews freeze wonderfully. Just take any of these options out of the freeze and put in fridge to defrost. Heat in microwave and garnish with some olive oils and herbs and grated cheese.

You may also want to purchase a cooler and some icepacks. In the case of power outage, or before a storm that might knock out the power, you can transfer all your prepared meals to the cooler, and because *they're already cooked, you have nutritious, safe foods to eat* cold.

Your frozen meals will stay cold longer in your freezer so those will be available too in the case of a power loss. All of this will help you avoid eating processed foods or having to go to the grocery store in these types of unexpected situations.

Conclusion

I hope this short introduction to the harm ultra-processed foods and drinks cause will help you being removing these substances from your life. Through trillions of dollars in advertising and marketing, we've been made to think that ultra-processed foods are a necessary part of life because they're "convenient" and because they're "healthy" according to our own national nutrition policy and most conventional advice about "healthy" eating.

These substances are toxic; they are not food.

Remember, don't be fooled by the rhetoric that a "calorie is a calorie." That's pure nonsense because the body doesn't recognize calories at any level or in any way. We cannot exercise our way out of a toxic diet that's been inflicted on us since the middle of the twentieth-century.

It's made trillions in profits for many companies, but this toxic diet of ultra-processed foods and sugar has caused widespread chronic metabolic diseases and conditions including obesity, Type 2 diabetes, hypertension, cardiovascular disease, dementia and more.

Ultra-processed foods and drinks are incredibly addictive because they're designed and manufactured to be addictive.

The companies who make them know this perfectly well. We must see ultra-processed foods and drinks as the descendants of the tobacco industry—and historically, the same industry. Addiction is the product—it's just the substance that has changed.

Finally, don't believe for a moment that you can't cook and make *incredible* meals at home. We're told constantly, both directly and indirectly, that it's just too complicated to cook and/or that we don't have enough time, or that we don't know what we're doing in the kitchen, etc.

These things aren't true—even if you've never cooked. We all understand food and we know a lot about food, even if we don't realize it. If you do **batch prep** (all the cutting and prep of the food) and **batch cooking**, you can prepare an entire week of meals in two hours—that's it—*two hours*. As your cutting and organization skills improve, it can take less time.

The key to eliminating ultra-processed foods and drinks from you life is *not having them in the house*. The second key is having a wide variety of meals that you can just pull together *quickly* by choosing the meat, poultry fish, vegetables, salad greens, and cooked grains you want.

You can assemble dinner in a matter of minutes for an entire family because everything is all there and prepared in your fridge.

This means dinner is a matter of getting a plate, which is very helpful if family members are on different schedules. Dinner plates can be filled with gorgeous foods warmed in the microwave or eaten cold during hot weather.

Nothing beats the flavor of whole and natural and real foods. It will take some time for your taste buds to recover from being overwhelmed by ultra-processed foods and drinks and sugar, but they will. As this happens, the cravings diminish considerably and become easier to manage.

These cravings may never disappear entirely; however, once you're blood sugar and insulin levels are more stable in response to a diet of whole and real foods that the human body recognizes and metabolizes properly, signaling satiety through the hormone leptin properly again, you'll find that the cravings are not nearly as intense.

Intense food cravings are very often sign of blood sugar and insulin problems, not lack of willpower—conditions caused and driven by foods that rapidly metabolize into sugar—ultra-processed foods and drinks and sugar in all forms.

Finally, remember this is a process; perfection is not the goal. Take the time you need to remove the ultra-processed foods and drinks and sugar from your diet, begin buying the foods listed in the staples section of this guide, and start preparing and cooking food using the batch method rather than trying to create complex meals from scratch each night.

These steps may mean you're about to make many changes in your eating and habits; take the time you need because doing these steps will transform your life and your health.

Printed in Great Britain
by Amazon

27844398R00065